]

To Joan,
with great affection,
  Enrique & Vilma
7/13

BRAIN SAFARI

SICK CHILDREN

SICK BRAINS

AND OTHER MALADIES

BY

Dan E. Keys

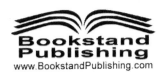
Bookstand
Publishing
www.BookstandPublishing.com

Published by
Bookstand Publishing
Morgan Hill, CA 95037
3865_7

ISBN 978-1-61863-420-7

Printed in the United States of America

Cover illustration: *The Doctor*, an oil painting by Sir Luke Fildes
(1843-1927). © Tate Museum, London, U.K.
(Reproduced with permission from Tate Images.)

PREFACE

When I left my native Costa Rica for the United States in 1955, I knew I would not return to live in that paradisiac, small country of gentle people, green mountains and beautiful songbirds. I was only eighteen and the passport to my future was a one-year scholarship as an exchange foreign student at Wesleyan University in Middletown, Connecticut. My goal was to study biochemistry. What I didn't know at the time is that I was destined to become a physician.

Medicine was not my first or even my second choice as a career. It was not seriously considered on my career list until my senior year in college in Ada, Oklahoma. I worked and lived in a small hospital and clinic run by a general practitioner, who decided I should go to medical school. I would have preferred to spend the rest of my life working in a laboratory and expected to be denied admission to medical school. Every objection I could think of such as, "no foreign student has been accepted before", "I have no money to pay for tuition" and "medicine is not my cup of tea", all fell by the wayside when I was admitted to the University of Oklahoma College of Medicine in 1959. An oil magnate and philanthropist offered to cover my tuition ($600 per semester in those days). To pay for my other expenses, I worked at night at the University Hospital clinical laboratories, while I caught up with my lack of sleep during the day in class. At the graduation ceremony I received the award for the best doctor-patient relationship, probably my greatest honor.

A rotating internship followed at Gorgas Hospital (1963-1964) in the Panama Canal Zone and fellowships in pediatrics (1964-1967) and neurology (1972-1975) at Mayo Clinic in Rochester, Minnesota. I became a pediatric neurologist, following the footsteps of my friend and mentor, Manuel R. Gomez. Since I could not see myself charging money for helping people, I chose academic medicine and spent the rest of my professional career in medical centers in Iowa (1975-1979), Virginia (1979-1991) and Kansas (1991-1996), except for a six-year period (1996-2002) organizing a pediatric neurology training program in the Middle East.

If I had to choose a motto for my life, this would be *Docendo Discimus*, which means "we learn by teaching". Teaching medical students and residents has been an enjoyable experience for me and I am certain that I have learned more from them than they have from me.

After my retirement from academic medicine in 2002, the next six years were spent writing a biography of Samuel Taylor Darling, an American pathologist who worked in Panama during the years of the construction of the canal (1904-1914). Darling discovered histoplasmosis in 1906, an important fungal disease. Writing Darling's biography was hard work but satisfying, even if the book did not sell more than a hundred copies. This was followed by another book about the American medical practice in Panama during the canal enterprise.

Darling's contributions to the sanitation of Panama made possible the successful construction of the Panama Canal. This theme appears repeatedly throughout this book, not with the purpose of boring the reader, but to emphasize the important role that this indefatigable pathologist and parasitologist played in the American engineering enterprise.

As a courtesy member of the Department of History and Philosophy of Medicine at the Kansas University Medical Center, under the leadership of Dr. Christopher Crenner, and of the Department of Pediatrics, under the leadership of Dr. Chet Johnson, I also contributed articles in Spanish on the medical history of Panama for the *Revista Cultural La Lotería* in Panama. One of these was entitled, "Clara Maass, la fiebre amarilla y el consentimiento informado [Clara Maass, yellow fever and informed consent]," and garnered an award as the best article in science or medicine published that year in *La Lotería* with an unexpected cash bonus of $1,000.

I had not previously considered writing about interesting patients I had seen in the past fifty years of medical practice for several reasons. Although Richard Selzer, Oliver Sacks and Atul Gawande have been successful as medical writers, few others have been able to do this well. That is, until a colleague at one of our meetings at the Clendening History of Medicine Library at the Kansas University Medical Center suggested that a book describing some of the interesting cases I had experienced in the past would be interesting. At least I now know there will be one person interested in reading this book.

Personal memoirs is not a popular genre and, therefore, no specific format has been predominant. I have selected short case vignettes and added pertinent or interesting explanatory material intended for both professional and non-professional readers, as well as a few bibliographic references when necessary at the end of each piece.

Colleagues who already know most of what I describe in this book may find it uninteresting or even differ or disagree with me on certain points. Hopefully, the majority of non-medical readers may find this book interesting and learn something about the world of pediatrics, tropical medicine and pediatric neurology. Any factual errors and misinterpretations are my sole responsibility. Names, places and clinical details have been altered in an effort to preserve the identity and privacy of the patients. Otherwise, all of the cases described are taken from true life, as strange as some of these may seem.

I wish to acknowledge my sincere gratitude to those who have read the manuscript and made helpful suggestions. I am especially indebted to Fred and Grace Holmes, whose vast experience and wisdom in medical matters I trust and value.

The use of a pseudonym is a matter of vanity. My complete name is Danilo Enrique Antonio de Jesús Chaves Carballo. The first four were given to me by well-meaning relatives, while Enrique was my father's name. He was born on July 14 and, according to the Catholic almanac, that is Enrique Emperador's (Henry the Emperor) day. The last two names are the paternal (Chaves) and maternal (Carballo) last names, usually hyphenated, since both together are not commonly used in English. The pseudonym consists of my real first name Dan (Danilo), the middle initial stands for Enrique and the last name is Chaves, which means "keys" in English.

Although my original plans did not include becoming a physician, I have accepted my given task and carried it out to the best of my abilities. Above all, I have tried to treat all my patients with respect and compassion. To them, I am grateful for the confidence they and their parents have placed in me.

Dan E. Keys
(Enrique Chaves-Carballo, M.D.)
Kansas City, Kansas

DEDICATION

To the sick children who taught me so much

and to those who care for them with love.

Contents

Cover Illustration   iv
Preface   v
Dedication   ix

I   **SICK CHILDREN**

1.   Reye and I   3

2.   My little boy blue   13

3.   Münchhausen   17

4.   Chemical autopsy   21

5.   Hemorrhagic shock   27

6.   Eating dirt   31

7.   Eating Jell-O®   35

II   **TROPICAL MALADIES**

8.   Fer-de-lance   41

9.   Yellow membrane   45

10.   Toxoplasmosis   51

11.   Yellow fever   59

12.   Germ of laziness   71

13.   Tuberculosis vaccine   75

14.   Mighty mites   81

15.   Neck maggots   85

16.   Moon children   89

17.   Head lice   93

18.   Malaria   97

III   SICK BRAINS

19.   Migraine   103

20.   Concussion   107

21.   Playing 'possum   111

22.   Status epilepticus   117

23.   Brain death   121

24.   Raggedy Ann   125

25.   Brown urine   129

26.   Cannibalism   135

27.   Hand movements   139

28.	Heatstroke	143
29.	Wear-and-tear pigments	147
30.	Red lobster	151
31.	Vertigo	157
32.	Muscle weakness	165
33.	Autism	169
34.	Startle disease	173
35.	Miracle doctor	177
IV	**OTHER MALADIES**	
36.	Life as an intern	183
37.	Hair biopsies	189
38.	Urine acids	193
39.	Familiar footsteps	199
40.	Pregnant frogs	203
41.	Libraries and books	207
42.	Medical writing	215

43. Expert witness   219

44. EMI scan   227

45. CNS   231

46. Dendrites and spines   235

Index   247

I

SICK CHILDREN

1

REYE AND I

Douglas Reye (1912-1977), a pathologist at the Royal Alexandra Hospital for Children in Sydney, Australia, published in 1963 in *Lancet*, a leading British medical journal, an epoch-making article entitled, "Acute encephalopathy and fatty degeneration of the viscera." Initially there was little to suggest that this report of twenty-one cases of brain swelling and fatty liver in children would become one of the most cited articles for the next thirty years.

George Johnson, a co-resident with me in pediatrics, also identified in 1963 sixteen cases of a fatal encephalitis among children in North Carolina similar clinically and pathologically to the cases in Australia. Because of the almost simultaneous descriptions of the syndrome by Reye and Johnson, the designation of Reye-Johnson syndrome was proposed but, unfortunately, without much support from subsequent authors.

Douglas Reye was a retiring, quiet man who went about his business in a methodical and unassuming manner. His entire professional career was spent at the same hospital and his death followed his retirement by only a few days. He only had a few publications to his credit prior to the description (along with his colleagues Graeme Morgan and James Baral) of what thereafter would be known as Reye syndrome. His main interests, aside from pathology, were working in his garden and driving vintage motorcars.

His colleagues described him as a quiet and competent worker, perhaps not prepared for the fame that would follow him after his publication in *Lancet*.

At first, no one was sure how to pronounce his name. Some would say "Righ" while others said his name meant "kings" or "*reyes*" in Spanish and, therefore, should be pronounced as "Ray." Finally, he clarified the confusion and explained that his name rhymed with "eye," and that inquiries about the correct pronunciation of his name were "much ado about nothing."

The importance of Reye's pathological description was the recognition at a microscopic level that the fatty appearance of the liver in his cases was different from that of typical alcoholic fatty liver. In the latter instance, the fat droplets in the hepatic cells were large and variable in size (fatty infiltration), while in the former these were all uniformly small or microdroplets (fatty degeneration). Only a few other conditions had been described with this kind of small droplet fatty degeneration and these were intoxications caused by aflatoxins (a potent toxin derived from the fungus *Aspergillus flavus*, which may contaminate cereals such as wheat, hay or rice), fatty liver of pregnancy and rare genetic metabolic diseases (also known as inborn errors of metabolism) affecting fatty oxidation and now known to be mitochondrial disorders with daunting names such as medium-chain acyl-CoA dehydrogenase deficiency (MCAD) and ornithine transcarbamylase deficiency (OTC). Another important finding in Reye's patients was increased blood ammonia levels (hyperammonemia) reflecting liver damage.

Not long after Reye's publication appeared in *Lancet*, similar cases were reported in the medical literature from other countries. Both physicians and the public began to ask: "Is this a new disease?"; "What causes it?"; "Is it an infection or a toxic reaction?"; but no one appeared to have any definitive answers. Surveillance studies by the Communicable Disease Center (CDC), as it was known then, showed that cases in the United States appeared mostly between December and April, affected mainly younger persons between the ages of 11 and 18 years, and that the illness was associated or, more accurately, followed influenza type B infections. More and more cases appeared so that before long over a thousand cases had been reported worldwide. Reye syndrome became the most common cause of acute encephalopathy among children in the United States in the 1960s and 1970s.

The clinical presentation was fairly uniform and predictable. The child would have a prodromal (preceding) illness characterized by fever, malaise and respiratory symptoms such as cough, or a gastroenteritis with diarrhea, about two or three weeks before the neurological presentation. The second phase appeared with repeated (protracted) vomiting and within hours or a few days, the child would become unresponsive and lapse into coma. Although in those days imaging of the brain was not possible since computed tomography (CT) and magnetic resonance imaging (MRI) had not been fully developed, autopsy studies showed that the coma resulted from brain swelling or edema. The swelling was potentially reversible and the patient was intubated, hyperventilated and given mannitol, an osmodiuretic, to try to reduce the brain swelling. After a few days, the child would recover apparently unharmed or, in about a third of the cases, die from herniation of the brain and injury to the brainstem where the centers that sustain life are located. The emotional trauma to both doctors and family members of the victims was incalculable, as could be expected from seeing a healthy child or adolescent suddenly go into coma and not survive.

As a young resident then, I participated in the diagnosis, care and pathological examination of many cases of Reye syndrome. Was there anything more we could do for these patients? Why was the etiology still a mystery? No one seemed to have any answers. At that point, I decided I would do research in Reye syndrome, although I had no idea how or where to start. An intuitive approach was to see how many cases had been seen at Mayo Clinic and examine in detail the medical records for possible clues. In order to find cases that may have been seen even prior to Reye's publication, a study was made of any cases with the diagnoses of coma, fatty liver, brain edema, acute encephalopathy, encephalitis and even toxic encephalopathy. The unique and excellent record-keeping system at Mayo facilitated this investigation and soon I was given a list of several hundred patients with one or more of these diagnoses. Each chart required detailed review and a form was devised to record all pertinent data on each patient, including name, age, sex, address, symptoms, examination, laboratory studies, treatment, etc. Several hours were spent delving on each medical chart to extract all the information needed. After almost a year, I had reviewed every possible case of Reye syndrome seen in Rochester, Minnesota.

The study yielded information on seventeen patients, some of whom had been seen even before Reye had recognized the new entity. The study was published as a leading article in the *Mayo Clinic Proceedings* and attracted some interest because it showed that Reye syndrome was not entirely a new disease. Reye syndrome had been present before 1963 but had not been recognized by clinicians or pathologists. Hence the genius of Douglas Reye, who first brought it to the attention of the world.

At this point, no one had any good ideas what could cause the brain swelling or the fatty degeneration of the liver in Reye syndrome. The prodromal influenza type B infection several weeks before the onset of vomiting and coma and the negative viral cultures of brain and liver samples negated the possibility that these pathological changes were due to direct damage from an infection. A more plausible explanation was that these were caused by some toxic agent or poison. I read avidly all publications about Reye syndrome but found no convincing answers.

During my third year as a neurology resident, I was given permission to spend at least six months doing basic research on Reye syndrome. I was fortunate to find support from Ralph D. Ellefson, Mayo's expert in lipid disorders, for my research project. Dr. Ellefson, a kind and sympathetic gentleman, found a corner in his laboratory and assigned Gayle Scanlon, one of his technicians, to teach me how to analyze lipids in tissue samples. By this time I had collected more than a dozen tissue samples from children who had died of Reye syndrome and kept these frozen at about 18 degrees centigrade below zero (-18° C) to assure the lipid components would not degrade from heat or exposure to air. Since my first passions had been biology and chemistry, I was now in complete heaven as a research fellow in Ellefson's laboratory.

Aflatoxin is one of the world's most potent toxins. It was calculated that as little as one microgram (one thousandth of a gram) was sufficient to kill a person. Exposure to this toxin had been reported from contaminated rice in Asia and death occurred from damage to the liver. Aflatoxin surveillance in the United States had failed to show any significant contamination of cereals and, therefore, aflatoxin intoxication was not deemed to be a significant public health problem in this country. Since I had a good number of liver samples and found an old ultraviolet spectrometer still in good working condition in the laboratory (thanks to Mayo's excellent medical and laboratory equipment maintenance team), I proceeded to analyze the tissues for aflatoxins. The initial testing was mainly a qualitative analysis based on the fact that aflatoxin B (the main culprit) is fluorescent when placed under ultraviolet light. The toxin was extracted with appropriate solvents and, to my surprise, one liver sample had a positive fluorescence for aflatoxin B. A more specific quantitative method was devised to measure the amount of toxin per gram of tissue using as a standard pure aflatoxin purchased from a biological supply company. Knowing that aflatoxin was one of the most potent toxins did not seem to cause me much concern, although I was careful to handle the chemical with protective gloves. However, none of the other liver samples showed the presence of aflatoxin B. The findings were published in an article in the *Mayo Clinic Proceedings* and, although it generated some interest, it did not clarify the etiology in the majority of cases of Reye syndrome.

The next step in the research plan was to analyze and identify more specifically the lipids responsible for the fatty degeneration in Reye syndrome. The laboratory techniques for lipid analyses at the time were rather crude and laborious. A small piece of liver was weighed in an analytical balance up to the nearest ten-thousandth of a gram (0.0001 gram). The tissue was then ground with a mortar and pestle cooled by surrounding ice and extracted with a mixture of methyl alcohol and chloroform. After extraction of the lipids, the solvents were evaporated with nitrogen gas (to avoid any exposure to oxygen) until completely dry and the residue once again weighed accurately. The lipids were then redissolved in an exactly measured amount of chloroform/methanol and placed in a spot on pure silica gel dried on glass plates for thin-layer chromatography. Chromatography was the time-honored technique used for separating a mixture of similar compounds by the capillary action of solvents moving in a plate or column of silica gel. I learned how to make the thin-layer chromatography plates using purified silica imported from Germany and, after what appeared to be hundreds of failed attempts until ready, started to separate and identify the lipid components in the liver samples. The plates were placed in glass chambers resting on the bottom immersed in a mixture of lipid solvents. The capillary action of the solvents on the silica gel separated the lipids into different components: triglycerides, phospholipids, fatty acids and cholesterol, using purified commercial standards in adjacent lanes for comparison. Each separated group of lipids was then scraped off the plates, extracted once again with appropriate solvents and then measured by standard spectrophotometric methods for more accurate quantitative results. Tissue phospholipids were more difficult to measure, but Dr. Ellefson had devised a good reproducible method that worked well enough for the study. After comparison of the results obtained and comparison with control tissue samples from normal liver, representing countless hours in the laboratory, nothing of note was found and all that could be said is that the lipid in the liver was mainly composed of triglycerides, something which had been suspected all along.

Almost a year after this "fishing expedition" in the laboratory in my quest to clarify the etiology of Reye syndrome, I had little to show. If I ask myself today would I have done anything differently or pursued a different direction for my research, the answer is still categorically "no!" The time spent in the laboratory investigating Reye syndrome remains one of my most cherished experiences and I am proud of the work I did, for I enjoyed every minute of it.

By now, there was a strong suspicion that liver degeneration in Reye syndrome was the result of damage to the mitochondria, small cell organelles where the energy that cells need is produced by oxidation of fatty acids. One of the candidate toxins was aspirin and animal experiments suggested that aspirin could cause something similar to Reye syndrome in rats. Epidemiological studies in the United States showed statistical evidence that children with Reye syndrome had been given aspirin more frequently than those who did not. Based on what I still consider a major blunder by public health authorities, a warning was widely circulated implicating a higher risk of Reye syndrome in children given aspirin.

The evidence against aspirin contributing to the cause of Reye syndrome was the fact that in many Asian and Latin American countries, aspirin continued to be used and yet the incidence of Reye syndrome appeared to wane as decades passed. As a sign of protest, my wife and I continued to give aspirin to our children, convinced that it had nothing to do with Reye syndrome.

Reye syndrome eventually almost disappeared and today most medical students and residents have not seen or even heard of Reye syndrome. Rarely, a child may present with brain swelling and damage to the liver but the diagnosis is usually one of the other mitochondrial disorders mentioned above.

Although I never had the privilege of meeting or hearing Douglas Reye at a medical meeting, to me he is like an old friend and I have long admired his talent as a pediatric pathologist. His observational skills, as well as his humble personality, remain an inspiration. As to Reye syndrome, I have much respect for this merciless killer of children, as I saw the victims and their families suffer immensely. This foe remained victorious in all attempts made to decipher the enigma of its predilection for the brain and liver of children. All I can say at this point is that I rejoice it no longer wreaks havoc and decimates children around the world.

Chaves-Carballo E, Gomez MR, Sharbrough FW: Encephalopathy and fatty infiltration of the viscera (Reye-Johnson syndrome). A 17-year experience. *Mayo Clinic Proceedings* 1975; 50: 209-15.

Chaves-Carballo E, Ellefson RD, Gomez MR: An aflatoxin in the liver of patient with Reye-Johnson syndrome. *Mayo Clinic Proceedings* 1976; 51: 48-50.

Chaves-Carballo E: Douglas Reye. In *The Founders of Child Neurology*. Ashwal S (ed), San Francisco: Norman Publishing, 1990; 826-30.

Reye RDK, Morgan G, Baral J: Encephalopathy and fatty degeneration of the viscera: A disease entity in childhood. *Lancet* 1963; 2: 749-52.

Johnson GM, Scurletis TD, Carroll NB: A study of sixteen fatal cases of encephalitis-like disease in North Carolina children. *North Carolina Medical Journal* 1963; 24: 464-473.

2

MY LITTLE BOY BLUE

Most doctors remember a unique patient or circumstance as especially difficult or trying. For a surgeon it might be a case complicated by unexpected bleeding during the operation. For an anesthesiologist it might be the sudden rise of core temperature indicating the catastrophic advent of malignant hyperthermia. Or for a neonatalogist it may be the realization that further efforts to resuscitate a twenty-four-week premature infant are no longer justified and the time has come to leave things alone. These and many other similar situations remind doctors of their limitations but also may engender heroic efforts that sometimes, although only rarely, turn the tide and bring back a life from the jaws of death. Occasionally there may be a patient who taxes our patience, ingenuity and ability to decipher a mysterious illness. Such was the case with "my little boy blue."

I call Bryan "my little boy blue" because one afternoon, as I walked into his room for my daily rounds at a children's hospital, the five-year-old turned blue and had no apparent cardiorespiratory problems to explain the discoloration of his skin. A light bulb suddenly went off in my head that clearly spelled *methemoglobinemia* and I ran down from the fifth floor to the pharmacy in the basement and requested urgently for a vial of methylene blue, which I promptly administered intravenously to the youngster. He immediately turned pink and went on about his business as if nothing unusual had happened.

But something important *had* happened in his blood. Hemoglobin is the complex protein that carries oxygen in our blood as oxyhemoglobin and makes it look red. The oxygen may be displaced or consumed so that the blood and, hence the skin, turns blue or cyanotic. Certain toxic substances such as nitrites in contaminated water, can also do this and convert the oxyhemoglobin into methemoglobin, turning the color of the skin a grayish blue. Although painless, methemoglobinemia results in deprivation of oxygen to vital organs that need it and consequent irreparable damage. Time is of the essence and therefore my haste in obtaining the antidote methylene blue.

My young patient would repeat this chameleon-like act many times in the ensuing months. Every test we did to elucidate the etiology of his repeated bouts of methemoglobinemia were fruitless. I took samples of Bryan's blood, urine and feces to my laboratory and tested them for any possible offending substance with uniformly negative results. Eventually, administration of methylene blue did not reverse the discoloration and we had to resort to exchange transfusions. This required ten or more pints of blood to replace Bryan's own defective blood and this was done in the intensive care unit manually with a catheter inserted into a large vein and a 30 cc. syringe was used to extract "bad" blood and infuse "good" blood. The cost of this and many other hospital expenses reached over a million dollars during the year Bryan remained hospitalized. Consultations with infectious diseases, gastroenterology, hematology, cardiology and every other subspecialty in the hospital, failed to unravel the mystery and I remained the primary physician, in charge of a "riddle, wrapped in a mystery, inside an enigma," to paraphrase Churchill's description of Russia.

In addition to methemoglobinemia, Bryan also had episodes of gagging, vomiting, seizures, and whatever else one might find in a textbook of pediatrics—all unexplained or at least poorly understood. A gastrointestinal motility study showed slow peristalsis but a trial of erythromycin did not improve his condition. Treatment with anticonvulsants also made no difference. Our inability to make a specific diagnosis eventually led to a dangerous path. Nurses began to whisper in my ear that his mother never left the bedside and this was one of the characteristics of *münchhausen by proxy* syndrome (mothers who purposefully make their children sick so they can get attention from the doctors and nurses). Although I had included this in my differential diagnoses at the beginning, I had convinced myself that it was not possible and every attempt to uncover a toxin or poison in the laboratory had proved negative. How was it possible to accuse someone without evidence of an offending weapon? I had seen a fair number of children who had been victims of münchhausen by proxy, but refused to accept this as an explanation for Bryan's unresolved problems. The parents had faith in me that I would cure their son and I had faith in them that they truly cared for him.

One day, while I was away on leave, my little boy blue turned blue for the last time. Bryan was taken to the intensive care unit and during one more exchange transfusion, his body gave up and attempts at resuscitation for a long period of time were ineffective. The funeral was attended by hundreds, since everybody in the hospital knew my little boy blue. His mother selected a few doctors and relatives to place a red rose on Bryan's small casket. I wanted to find an excuse not to go because I had failed to keep Bryan alive, to know what ailed him. As I walked slowly and placed the flower over him, I thought about how brilliant the red rose was. If only we had found a way to transfer that vibrant red color to his own blood. But doctors are not magicians and only a magician could have done that.

3

MÜNCHHAUSEN

The mother was an attractive, slender, young woman with a brilliant smile that immediately generated tender feelings. Everyone was sympathetic to her plight. She had already lost one of her babies to sudden infant death syndrome (SIDS) and now a second infant, Joshua, was developing respiratory problems (apnea) when asleep at night.

Apnea, especially in premature infants, results when the brain stem is not sufficiently developed to keep respirations going as carbon dioxide concentrations increase in the blood and alert the respiratory center to continue breathing. These infants are sent home with apnea monitors so that apnea is detected and the parents can intervene when the infant stops breathing. This requires hospital personnel to instruct the mother how to give cardiorespiratory resuscitation (CPR) and prevent death or brain damage from low oxygen blood levels (hypoxia). It is not unusual for a family to have both apnea and SIDS in different babies. Presumably, the defective respiratory center may have a genetic basis.

After repeated hospitalizations, suspicions began to mount that the underlying problem might be münchhausen by proxy syndrome. The name of Baron Münchhausen (1720-1797) had become synonymous with "false and ridiculously exaggerated exploits" when a book (authored by someone else) described his adventures in Russia. The name first appeared in the medical literature in 1951 and was used to describe a patient who exaggerated or fabricated an illness as a means of becoming the center of attention from doctors and nurses. Twenty-five years later, a permutation, *münchhausen by proxy*, was introduced to describe a form of child abuse when a parent (usually the mother) deliberately harms, poisons or creates abnormal findings (such as blood in the urine) in a child. This situation usually results in diagnostic challenges and exaggerated attention from medical caregivers in hospitals.

As a pediatric neurologist over several decades, my confidence in the honesty and goodness of most parents has seldom waivered. I have seen too many dedicated and selfless parents protect and accompany their children through the ordeals of sickness and suffering. My faith in the goodness of human beings has remained unshaken through the years. But I have also seen the darker side of those who physically abuse children and have had the unenviable task of pronouncing dozens of such victims of *shaken-baby syndrome* as brain dead. The memories of x-rays showing broken ribs and long bones, as well as skull fractures, stand silently as irrefutable proof of the unlimited cruelty some human beings can perpetrate on defenseless children. Pediatricians consider themselves as advocates of vulnerable children and have the responsibility to report these cases to the proper authorities.

The investigations for repeated apnea in Joshua, our patient, included a video-EEG (a video-brain wave test), consisting of monitoring of the brain waves along with a video recording of the child's activity, and cardiac as well as respiratory monitoring throughout the day and night. Twenty-four hours later, we had been unable to capture or record any abnormality or apneic episodes and decided to discontinue this type of monitoring. After notifying the mother that we had concluded the test, we told her that the video recording apparatus would stay in the room until next morning but that it was turned off. The mother was unaware that the video had been left *on* on purpose.

During the night, Joshua's mother got up several times and approached the infant crib as if to check and make sure everything was fine. To our amazement, she then placed her hands on Joshua's neck and gently pressed until the baby could not breathe, triggering the apnea monitor. When the nurse responded to the alarm, the mother calmly reported that Joshua had stopped breathing and she had stimulated him to resume breathing. This was repeated several times during the night. Next morning, the video recording was removed from the room and reviewed. Our eyes could not believe what had transpired the night before and yet it was all there, in the video recording. Some of us experienced a feeling of nausea while others shook their heads in disbelief.

We returned and confronted the mother with the evidence and contacted the protective services, who took responsibility for the welfare of the infant and the mother was incarcerated pending review of the case and testimony from the medical witnesses. Once this process concluded, I felt relief that this sordid case was over. However, the astute defense attorney mounted an effective argument that the incriminating evidence had been obtained under false pretenses and without the mother's permission. The judge in this case ruled in favor of the mother and, to our dismay, the infant was returned to her care.

It is the moral obligation of child advocates to report child abuse. However, the responsibility of designating culpability in these cases rests wholly in the hands of the legal system. Civil liberties are important, for these are the basis for our rights to freedom of speech, religion and political preferences. However, I cannot agree with the freedom to protest at the funeral of a soldier or in front of an abortion clinic. I also disagree with the right of a motorcyclist not to wear a helmet or the right of anyone to possess an assault weapon. Our emergency departments are too busy attending the consequences of what to me are such irresponsible acts. We must not confuse freedom with anarchy. At times we are disappointed when someone we thought was culpable is found not guilty because of some technicality. In those cases we realize that the rules and laws must be followed explicitly for the legal system to be effective. However, when a defenseless child is returned to the care of the perpetrator who violated moral and social principles, as in this case, then the justice system has failed to protect the most vulnerable and defenseless of victims.

Olry R: Baron Münchhausen and the syndrome which bears his name: History of an endearing personage and of a strange medical disorder. *Vesalius* 2002; 8: 53-7.

4

CHEMICAL AUTOPSY

The mother had brought her three-month-old girl, Elizabeth, three times to the hospital Emergency Room because of vomiting and dehydration. The episodes had a sudden onset, usually preceded by what seemed a common prodromal illness, and were accompanied by upper respiratory symptoms and fever. Each time, Elizabeth was given intravenous fluids and sent home to recover from another "viral" infection or "flu-bug." On the third visit, however, the infant was now *in extremis* and did not survive despite all efforts to resuscitate her and restore her to normalcy. The discharge diagnosis was ALTE (Acute Life-Threatening Event), another euphemism for what at one time was also called near-miss SIDS (Sudden Infant Death Syndrome). The doctors use these acronyms to hide our ignorance about what has really happened and include modifiers such as idiopathic (unknown cause) and cryptogenic (undecipherable cause) to further disguise our ignorance.

The state laws stipulated that any infant who died unexpectedly must have an autopsy. At one time, autopsies were required as an effective teaching tool. John Cabot introduced nearly two hundred years ago the clinicopathological conference in the *Boston Medical & Surgical Journal*, precursor of the *New England Journal of Medicine*. The format required first a detailed presentation of the case history, examination and laboratory results and, if available, x-ray findings. An experienced clinician would then discuss the differential diagnosis and arrive at a final conclusion based on his knowledge and available information. The conference would then be handed over to the pathologist, who had the last word, and a description of the findings at autopsy (or at surgery, biopsy or specific laboratory test) would confirm or refute the diagnosis offered by the specialist. The teaching value of the clinicopathological conference, or CPC as it was usually called, was universally recognized and accepted.

The status of a teaching hospital at the time was not only related to the excellence and experience of its teachers, variety of teaching cases, depth and breadth of its medical library, and sophistication of its laboratory and radiological facilities, but also on the percentage or number of autopsies performed. The CPC served not only as a teaching tool for medical students and residents, but also pointed out faculty judgment errors that should have been avoided. Autopsies, however, gradually began to loose their lofty status as a sacred teaching exercise. During the transformation of medicine from a profession to a business, the value of an autopsy was misinterpreted as the "cost" of an autopsy. Since insurance carriers did not reimburse the hospital or the patient for an autopsy, this exercise no longer was "cost-effective," and slowly became obsolete unless, as in our case, a medicolegal aspect justified the performance of an autopsy.

The reluctance of family members of the deceased to have an autopsy performed was, in the past, not a major reason to desist from obtaining permission.

The first objection by the family was commonly based on the erroneous concept that the pathological examination would deform the appearance of the body (mainly the face). The second objection was the delay this would entail and the family was not willing to wait a day or two to take the body home.

During the three years I was a resident in pediatrics, I learned how to obtain permission for an autopsy and was not once refused. First of all, the family has to be approached with kindness and respect. The loss of a child, perhaps more than that of an adult, is heartrending. After clarification that the examination will be done with respect, that no vestiges will be apparent, and that there will be no undue delay in making the funeral arrangements, the main justification given is that the autopsy will clarify the cause of death and teach us how to recognize and treat this problem more readily in the future. Finally, as a teaching institution this hospital requires for autopsies to be done in as many of the children who have died, as a measure of its excellence. There is no room during this painful encounter for excuses, coercion or impatience. A good rapport with the family prior to the bad outcome may be of inestimable value in securing permission.

Autopsies are now seldom performed unless the situation becomes a medicolegal case. Modern genetic and neuroimaging tests often provide the final diagnosis without an autopsy. However, some pathologists will include in their examination what is now called a *chemical autopsy*. This examination is similar to the expanded newborn screening done soon after the birth of an infant.

Newborn screening consisted initially of testing for phenylketonuria (PKU), one of the most common causes of mental retardation. PKU, if identified and treated early by dietary elimination of phenylalanine, will prevent damage to the brain. A second important screening test was for hypothyroidism, which no longer is a major cause of mental retardation, thanks to the universal use of iodized salt. Other biochemical tests in the newborn were screening for homocystinuria, mucopolysaccharidoses and galactosemia, using colorimetric qualitative tests on random urine samples. Thus, five metabolic disorders could be readily screened in the 1950s from a single urine sample.

Automation of more sophisticated analytical apparatuses in the 1990s led to the introduction of mass screening utilizing mass spectrometry, also known as *tandem MS*. This powerful new technique allows for automated screening of more than forty congenital metabolic disorders (inborn errors of metabolism or IEM) in three hundred blood spot samples obtained by neonatal heel sticks and run in the laboratory overnight.

The cost-effectiveness of tandem MS was questioned at first. The incidence of inborn errors of metabolism ranges from 1:10,000 births (as in PKU) to 1:300,000 in more rare disorders, while most of these disorders have a frequency of 1:100,000 births. However, there are more than eight hundred inborn errors of metabolism, of which about forty can be readily tested by tandem-MS. The incidence of IEM then increases from 1:100,000 to about 1:2,500, identifiable with a single blood-spot sample. The arithmetic now indicates cost-effectiveness for newborn screening when compared to the cost to the state of treating and providing supporting services such as physical therapy, behavioral therapy, occupational therapy, speech/ language therapy and other modalities needed by an affected child for the remainder of his or her life.

A chemical autopsy is performed on a blood sample sent to a referral laboratory. The tandem-MS screening can be done at a cost of less than $100 ($41 at Mayo Medical Laboratories in 2009). The pathologist who sent the test was mainly guided by the finding at autopsy of a fatty liver, an infiltration of the liver cells by fat droplets sometimes seen in IEM. After a couple of weeks, the results showed that the infant had a rare IEM affecting the oxidation of fatty acids and probably responsible for her death. Furthermore, this was a potentially treatable condition if identified early and implementation of proper treatment with dietary supplements. After a considerable deliberation, the family sued the hospital and the case was settled out of court for an undisclosed sum.

Although monetary compensation to the family will not bring back their child, it is important that such children with rare disorders be identified and treated early. Dietary restrictions and avoidance of infection often may return the child to a normal life. Technological advances now facilitate the identification of rare disorders and physicians can no longer claim ignorance as an excuse for missing the diagnosis in similar cases.

Chace DH, DiPema JC, Mitchell BL, et al: Electrospray tandem mass spectrometry for analysis of acylcarnitines in dried postmortem blood specimens collected at autopsy from infants with unexplained cause of death. *Clinical Chemistry* 2001; 47: 1166-82.

Mayo Clinic. Mayo Medical Laboratories. 2009 Test
Catalog. CPT Code No. 81931 Postmortem Screening, Bile
and Blood Spots, p. 592.

5

HEMORRHAGIC SHOCK

The landmark article first appeared in the respected British journal *Lancet* in 1983. The authors had seen within the past year ten infants who presented with acute onset of fever, shock, watery diarrhea, severe hepatic and renal dysfunction and an encephalopathy. They thought that this was a new or previously unrecognized disorder.

Although I had not seen the report, one of my colleagues had and when Laurie, the first patient with similar symptoms, was admitted to our hospital pediatric intensive care unit, the clinical diagnosis was easily made. Laurie had been sick with fever and irritability for two days and then was found unresponsive and brought to the hospital in an ambulance. The rectal temperature was 107 degrees Fahrenheit (42 degrees Centigrade). Laurie stopped breathing and was intubated but suffered a cardiac arrest and her blood pressure was undetectable. She was resuscitated with adrenaline, bicarbonate, atropine, dopamine and fluids, as well as albumin. A bleeding disorder (coagulopathy) was detected and her platelet count was decreased (79,000 per cu mm). Prothrombin and partial thromboplastin times were prolonged and the presence of fibrin derivatives confirmed the presence of a disseminated intravascular coagulopathy (DIC). Liver function tests were abnormal (2,000 units per liter for AST) and renal function tests also showed abnormal function with a creatinine of 1.7 mg/deciliter, and the presence of albuminuria and hematuria was detected in the urine analysis. The clinical features were consistent with the cases reported in *Lancet* by Levin et al. Before the end of the decade, we had seen a total of nine cases and our experience was reported in the *American Journal of Diseases of Children*.

When I was asked to review a medicolegal case for the plaintiff, the features were clearly one of this disorder. The intensivists and neurologists had not recognized the disorder and failure to do so had resulted in moderately severe brain damage. Our previous experience with such cases facilitated the defense as an expert witness and the case was settled by the hospital, as usual, out of court.

A couple of years later Laurie, the child whom I had been following now in the clinic, presented with an acute illness and I referred her to the same hospital where she had been misdiagnosed. The hospital director became adamant and initially refused to admit her but then reconsidered when he realized that this would not be good public relations for the hospital.

I see my role as an expert witness is to disclose the truth and help whoever is right, either the plaintiff or the defense. Therefore, I will not accept participating in a case unless I have verified the facts and determined to my satisfaction which side is justified.

My first medicolegal case as an expert witness involved a general practitioner in a small rural town who had made a mistake and was tormented by the results. He was a good friend of the family and visited the child daily at home afterwards. The family, nevertheless, sued and although we were successful in defending his case in that it was not the result of negligence and that the doctor had acted as expected from a general practitioner in a rural area and not as a specialist from a tertiary medical center, he abandoned his practice and did not see any more patients for the rest of his life, as far as I know. An honest mistake had cost him his career and the town no longer counted with the services of a dedicated doctor. He suffered more emotional trauma than the child had in physical injuries. Such cases may sadly end up in suicide. Doctors have a high incidence of suicide and that is the price some pay for the privilege of serving others.

The best protection against malpractice demands is to establish a good rapport between the physician and patient. Establishing a trust between both parties helps to understand and forgive when a mistake has been made. But, as in this case, this was not enough and greedy plaintiffs may prefer to incriminate the doctor or hospital. Money can be a powerful incentive in these cases.

Although not common, cases of hemorrhagic shock and encephalopathy in children were seen more frequently. As our experience increased, the diagnostic criteria were modified to include younger patients. I was asked to serve as an expert witness in additional cases that had been missed or misdiagnosed. One of the defense attorneys, aware that the diagnostic criteria for hemorrhagic shock and encephalopathy had been changed over the years, tried to use this as a means to discredit the validity of the diagnosis. The rebuttal claimed that medicine is always evolving and new information requires revision of old concepts. This does not mean that previous concepts were wrong; it only means that medicine is a dynamic body of knowledge that is constantly changing to accommodate new truths.

More than thirty years later, the cause of hemorrhagic shock and encephalopathy remains unknown. As in heatstroke, the presence of a high body temperature may initiate a cascade of physiological events mediated by the release of inflammatory cytokines that, in turn, damage tissues, including liver and kidneys. The site of predominant injury appears to be in the lining (endothelial wall) of the bowel. Multiorgan failure and disseminated intravascular coagulopathy (DIC), along with shock, conspire together to produce this catastrophic illness. Early recognition and intervention to reverse shock and hemorrhage may stop the seemingly relentless progression toward death in these unfortunate children, but the chances for survival remain poor.

Chaves-Carballo E, Montes JE, Nelson B, et al: Hemorrhagic shock and encephalopathy. Clinical definition of a catastrophic syndrome in infants. *American Journal of Diseases in Children* 1990; 144: 1079-1082.

Levin M, Kay JDS, Gould JD, et al: Haemorrhagic shock and encephalopathy: A new syndrome with a high mortality in young children. *Lancet* 1983; 2: 64-7.

6

EATING DIRT

My first scientific publication almost fifty years ago presented seventeen children with lead poisoning and indicated that this problem was not rare in Panama. Twelve of the seventeen children had *pica*, an abnormal appetite for things not fit to eat. The most common complaints in these children were vomiting, convulsions, anorexia, weight loss, pallor and irritability. Ten of the children had ingested paint flakes or chips. Treatment by *chelation* (chemical binding of the offending agent) resulted in symptomatic improvement.

Lead poisoning or intoxication in children may account for behavioral and learning problems, including hyperactivity, poor memory and aggressive, antisocial and compulsive behavior. Public awareness of the deleterious consequences of lead poisoning has led to restrictions on the use of gasoline, paint, earthenware and toys containing lead. Lead screening has been implemented in vulnerable populations and the previous threshold for dangerous blood lead levels has been lowered from 10 to 5 µg per ml and now to 1 µg per ml.

The word pica has its origins in the Greek name for magpie, a bird related to crows and presumed to steal and hide all kinds of unlikely objects. Pica is not unusual in animal species such as camels, elephants and macaws, which may travel long distances to ingest clay and dirt thought to contain essential minerals. Pica is also known among pregnant women who may crave certain indulgences but also at times inappropriate ones. Finally, pica may not be that uncommon among toddlers who have learned to crawl and put into their mouths anything they can reach.

Lead poisoning can be recognized by the presence of radiopaque ingested paint chips and prominent lead lines in routine x-rays of the abdomen or long bones. Clues may also be found in the appearance of basophilic stippling (dark blue dots) in red blood cells, as well as changes in the appearance of red blood cells similar to those found in iron-deficiency anemia. Cultural practices such as darkening the eyes with *kohl* (containing lead and from which the name for alcohol is derived) in Arab and Indian populations, may increase the exposure to lead.

Our favorite cockatiel was found to have lead-paint chips in her stomach, probably due to her bad habit of scraping with her beak the white paint on the wires of her birdcage. Unfortunately, she didn't survive her pica and lead poisoning. This reminded me also of our childhood fascination playing with lead soldiers and jumping jacks without knowing then the dangers of lead exposure.

The toxicity of lead in the nervous system may lead to brain swelling when acute or to demyelination (destruction of myelin) when chronic. The former leads to vomiting and potentially lethal brain herniation, while the latter may result in painful neuropathies resembling the burning sensations in the limbs of diabetic patients.

All of the so-called heavy metals, including mercury, arsenic, beryllium, cadmium and lead, are toxic and exposure to humans must be carefully controlled. Mercury used to be common in household items such as thermometers. Its unusual chemical and physical properties attracted our interest as children, ignorant of its ability to sublimate and then penetrate our bodies through our nostrils as almost invisible pellets. Before Occupational Safety and Health Administration (OSHA) regulations, a mercury spill in the laboratory was simply handled with a small broom and scoop tray, recovering as much of the dispersing silvery glob back to the wide-mouth glass container.

Finally, returning to my first publication on lead poisoning in children, this was the first of many articles, abstracts and chapters that would follow in the ensuing decades. The long-held adage in academic medicine of "publish or perish" was so true and the rise from assistant to associate to full professor still depends much on such productivity. There is also something called *gusanillo* in Spanish, which means "little worm." This little worm is an invisible parasite that enters the body and lodges in the brain of unsuspecting subjects and programs them to publish and publish and publish. It doesn't demand any specific requirements for excellence. It consumes all your time and energy. There is no limit to the number of publications required to reach its point of satiety. In summary, it is like an insatiable pica that, similar to lead poisoning, poisons your brain and, as far as I know, there is no cure for this malady.

Guerra Millikan CR, Chaves Carballo E: Lead poisoning in children in Panama. *Archivos Médicos Panameños* 1964; 13: 70-4.

7

EATING JELL-O®

Little Michael was only six months old and was doing well developmentally. However, his mother insisted that whenever she gave him Jell-O® (which he liked very much), Michael would become lethargic and, on a couple of occasions, had difficulty waking him up. The story had components that suggested fabrication, but the mother insisted on its veracity.

Trying to think of a salomonic solution to this conundrum, I asked her to bring some of the Jell-O® she prepared and also a sample of urine after Michael had ingested the red gelatin. She complied eagerly to my request and within a few days she had delivered to my laboratory both specimens. The extraction for organic acids was simple and straightforward, using the usual solvents and then methylating the component acids for analysis by gas chromatography/mass spectrometry (GC/MS) with trimethylsilyl (TMS) derivatives. The Hewlett-Packard GC/MS apparatus was my pride and joy, even though it required for me to spend countless hours comparing manually the results obtained from each analysis (computerized databases were not yet readily available). I had no expectations that Michael's urine would provide us with any clues to help clarify his mother's observations.

The urine analysis, however, did show a very large amount of adipic acid, an organic acid commonly found in normal urine. Adipic is a six-carbon dicarboxylic acid mainly derived from dietary sources and not associated with any known disease. Its presence in the urine was not surprising but the very large amount (more than a hundred times the usual concentration), definitely was. The next step was to analyze the Jell-O$^®$ the mother had brought. Once again, to my surprise, this was also chock-full of adipic acid! But what did all this mean? All I knew then was that children like Jell-O$^®$ but older people don't. An old joke was about the tenant in a home for the elderly who refused to eat Jell-O$^®$ because he didn't want to eat something that shook more than he did.

The Society for the Study of Inborn Errors of Metabolism, to which I belonged, published a fine journal, the *Journal of Inherited Metabolic Diseases* (*JIMD*). Our medical library did not carry this journal but, fortunately, I had purchased a complete collection for my laboratory. In one of the *JIMD* issues, many years later, a similar case was described in a short report. However, the patient in that case was a 28-year-old woman and, although she was developmentally delayed, she did not have any neurological symptoms ascribable to adipic acid. A closely related condition, ethylmalonic-adipic aciduria, was well known but Michael's urine analysis had not shown any ethylmalonic acid—only adipic, thus effectively ruling out this condition.

The composition of Jell-O$^®$ listed in the package includes adipic acid as an ingredient for tartness, but its concentration is not given. The toxicity of adipic acid for humans is not clear. Data from rats suggest only a mild toxicity since the LD_{50} of adipic acid is about 3 grams per kilogram (that is, that much is lethal to half of the experimental rats). For a six-month-old infant who weighs approximately 7.5 kilograms, this is equivalent to about 20 grams of adipic acid—a very large amount, indeed!

One possible explanation for Michael's sensitivity to adipic acid may have been in the metabolic pathway used to metabolize adipic acid in his own mitochondria. This would require sending a tissue sample from skin or muscle to a specialized laboratory. In those days this type of testing was not available commercially and was usually done by a research laboratory by courtesy, which meant an indefinite period of time waiting and sometimes the sample would even become lost or never tested. The other investigative possibility was to put little Michael through a series of "loading" tests with pure adipic acid to measure how much he was able to tolerate without neurologic symptoms. Neither his mother nor myself was willing to do this.

At the end, the simplest solution was the obvious one: don't give Michael any more Jell-O®! And that was the end of that. As the old saying goes, "Prudence or discretion is the better part of valor".

Glick N, Fischer M: Adipic aciduria: a dietary artefact. *Journal of Inherited Metabolic Diseases* 1991; 14: 8.

II

TROPICAL

MALADIES

8

FER-DE-LANCE

The young girl, Imelda, was only ten years old and came from nearby María Chiquita, a village about fifteen miles from Coco Solo Hospital, an American hospital on the Atlantic side of the Panama Canal Zone. Imelda had gone out the backdoor of her home and in doing so, stepped on a fer-de-lance pit viper (*Bothrox atrox*), the most poisonous snake in Panama and responsible for more deaths than any other species. She was brought by ambulance to our Emergency Room, where I was on call that weekend.

A rapid evaluation showed that Imelda was already *in extremis*. She was poorly responsive to stimulation and her gums were oozing blood, indicating that the serpent's venom had already circulated into her brain and supporting systems. Two distinct fang marks on her left foot were already swollen and blue. Imelda's chances for survival appeared slim. The neurotoxins and hematotoxins contained in the venom had already wreaked havoc in her frail body. Not having any previous experience with snakebites and failing to recall any lectures on the subject during my training years, I called immediately Gorgas Hospital, the main hospital on the Pacific side, and asked for the specialist expert in snake envenomations, only to be told he was on leave and unavailable.

Young physicians have all experienced that "sinking" feeling of despair when control of a critical situation has been lost and the patient appears to be no longer salvageable. According to Sir William Osler, the physician must always be in control and divorce himself or herself from the emotional situation, lest his/her leadership role and ability to instill confidence be undermined. But physicians are human beings and, as much as they may try to hide their emotions behind an impassive face and measured responses, remain vulnerable to the suffering of others. The loss of any patient, particularly a child, is always heartrending and depressing.

Not knowing exactly how to proceed, but aware that the seconds and minutes were critical in this case, I rushed to the pharmacy, unlocked the entrance and opened the refrigerator, where five vials of antivenom were stored. The antiserum, also called Butantán serum because it was mainly obtained from the Butantán Institute in Brazil, was the only remedy available. I ran back to the Emergency Room and not knowing exactly the recommended dose to be given to a child, decided to give Imelda four of the vials intravenously and save the remaining one if there was no favorable response. Within thirty minutes, she began to respond better and the bleeding improved. After two hours I knew Imelda would survive and felt an immense sense of relief.

The conventional wisdom at the time, I found out later after searching in the *Index Medicus* for current references on treatment of snakebites, was that the antiserum was given according to weight, so that a child would receive much less than an adult in similar circumstances. However, my logic was different. The snake did not know if the victim was a child or an adult, and injected most of the venom in self-defense. This volume of venom, I reasoned, would be more concentrated in the circulation of a child than in an adult and, therefore, the child deserved a much larger dose of antiserum than an adult. If I were going to err in this case, I would rather do so on the excessive amount rather than on an insufficient dose. Imelda had only one chance to survive and I was not going to waste it.

After one week, the fortunate girl recovered enough to be discharged from our hospital and referred to orthopedics because the site of the snakebite had swollen excessively to the point that circulation to the foot could be impaired. A timely fasciotomy released the ligaments of the foot and circulation was restored. One month later, the family returned to see me and brought a pineapple as a token of gratitude. I accepted the gift wholeheartedly and tried to emulate Sir William Osler's dictum, but without success. It was impossible not to celebrate with the family the survival of their beautiful daughter.

Snakebites are responsible for many deaths around the world, particularly in places such as India and South America. The time-honored immediate treatment seen in Western movies, consisting of sucking the venom through the puncture wounds and placing a tourniquet proximal to the bite site to prevent the poison from circulating freely, is not only useless, but probably deleterious. At one time the Instituto Butantán was the only source of anti-venom, produced by harvesting antibodies from inoculated horses. The possibility of an anaphylactic reaction to horse serum was counteracted by the certain death that followed a bite from a pit viper.

Robert Grocott, a quiet but ingenious laboratory technician at Gorgas Hospital in Panama, had published a small but invaluable manual on the identification of poisonous snakes in Panama. He also had developed a silver stain used to facilitate the identification of fungi such as histoplasmosis in tissue sections. Grocott's reserved and humble personality belied the importance of these two major contributions he made to medical science.

Clodomiro Picado (also known as "Clorito") was the only true scientist Costa Rica had at the turn of the Twentieth Century. Clorito had studied immunology at the Pasteur Institute in Paris and local legend was that he was so brilliant that he had discovered penicillin before Fleming and also had found that ageing was the result of antibodies produced against vital organs. He returned to Costa Rica and established his laboratories at the San Juan de Dios Hospital in San José. Any snakebite victim who survived long enough to be brought to this hospital benefited from his knowledge about snakes. He also produced sufficient quantities of anti-venom to supply the needs of the hospital. I am proud to have in my collection the seven volumes of his research publications and consider him to be the most outstanding scientist Costa Rica has ever produced. Although he received no honors or awards from the government for his work during his lifetime, Clorito must have had the great satisfaction of saving more snakebite victims than any other person in Costa Rica. I wondered how many pineapples he must have received from grateful patients.

Grocott RG: *Poisonous Snakes in Panama*. Canal Zone: Mt. Hope Press, 1958.

Picado Twight C: *Obras Completas* (vol 1-7), Cartago: Editorial Tecnológica de Costa Rica, 1988.

9

YELLOW MEMBRANE

The introduction of vaccination to protect from smallpox by Jenner in 1796 represents a major paradigm shift in the protection of humans from infectious diseases. Jenner's observations that milkmaids appeared to be resistant to acquiring smallpox and that often they experienced a milder form of the disease called cowpox, led to his successful inoculation of a child with cowpox.

This epochal event in the history of medicine was not obstructed by requirements of approval by an institutional review board or need for informed consent, whether written or not. The ethics of human experimentation did not come to the forefront until the Nuremberg trials in 1964 and the first modern use of written informed consent was introduced in 1900 by Walter Reed in his experiments to prove that yellow fever was transmitted by contaminated mosquitoes. Jenner would never obtain approval today for his experimental use of a child. Most probably, he would be stripped of his medical license and condemned for putting a child's life at risk.

Jenner's successful inoculation with an attenuated microorganism opened the way for protection of susceptible populations by mass immunization. The disappearance of smallpox and the near-eradication of other dreadful childhood diseases such as poliomyelitis were a direct result of Jenner's improbable intuition. It is almost impossible to accurately calculate the number of children who have been saved from the three apocalyptic horsemen, diphtheria, pertussis (whooping fever) and tetanus, by DPT immunization. Unfortunately, ignorance and prejudice have undermined this herd immunity and outbreaks of whooping cough and measles have recently emerged among unvaccinated children.

While learning and training as a medical student and resident in pediatrics and neurology in the United States, I never saw a case of diphtheria, whooping cough or tetanus in a child. An adult with tetanus was hospitalized in Minnesota but I was not involved in his care and only remember that he was in a quiet, dark room, while heavily sedated. Thus, I was unprepared and quite ignorant about childhood infectious diseases still present in underdeveloped countries. After finishing medical school, I elected to do my rotating internship at Gorgas Hospital in Panama in 1963 and after completing my pediatric training, returned to Panama in 1967 to work as a pediatrician.

My first patient as an intern at Gorgas Hospital was a man from the leper colony at Palo Seco. Leprosy was certainly not among the rare and exotic diseases I saw in the United States. Thanks to the expertise of Dr. Cedeño, who had obtained spectacular results with treatment of leprosy lesions with chaulmoogra oil, we all learned much about this interesting disease of antiquity caused by Hansen's bacillus. The bacillus prefers to proliferate in tissues with less circulation and warmth, such as nose, fingers and toes, resulting in their destruction and grotesque appearance. This was also the first and only case I have seen of amyloidosis of the kidneys, a possibly fatal complication of leprosy.

As a pediatrician, I began to see children with infectious diseases I had not seen before during my years of training. Whooping cough was not uncommon and the diagnosis was easily made clinically with the unmistakable "barking" cough. Tetanus was also commonly seen but mostly in neonates delivered by midwives who had cut the umbilical cord with contaminated scissors or razor blades. Chickenpox and measles were also common and searching for that single, skin first blister with the purulent exudate and surrounding redness required the patience and persistence of a Sherlock Holmes, including the magnifying glass which I always carried in my pocket but without the stereotyped thinking cap. Measles was another childhood illness that offered little if any diagnostic challenge due to the unmistakable conjunctival hyperemia (eye redness) and persistent cough (often pneumonia). But the most feared childhood illness was diphtheria.

The diagnosis was not suspected early in the course of the illness. Not until breathing became laborious and inspection of the nasal passages or pharynx revealed the presence of the unmistakable yellow, thick membrane adhering to the mucosal surfaces, confirmed the dreadful diagnosis. At the time, intubation and ventilator support were not available options in our hospital and tracheotomy was a last-ditch procedure with seldom any good results. Treatment consisted of giving the child diphtheria antitoxin and this worked surprisingly well. A child who seemed to be suffocating because the upper airway was severely compromised by the diphtheritic membrane, would respond within twenty four hours and recovery was then assured.

Thus, Magali, a sprite eight-year-old Panamanian girl, was admitted with diphtheria, treated with antitoxin and recovered completely. She returned home to her grateful parents. Less than a year later, Magali returned very sick, her breathing compromised and near death. Examination of her throat revealed the thick, angry, yellow membrane of diphtheria! How could this be?, I asked myself incredulously. Magali had had diphtheria already and that exposure meant that she had developed a natural immunity to the Loeffler's bacillus, *Corynebacterium diphtheriae*.

Already sensing Magali's imminent death, I called Dr. Rodolfo Young, one of the world's experts in tuberculosis and chest diseases (Dr. Young would later become dean of the medical school at the University of Panama). He came immediately and aware of the dire situation, ordered for the patient to be taken to the operating room, where he inserted an endoscope in an effort to dislodge the diphtheritic membrane and attempt to perform a tracheotomy. We both felt numb and defeated as this promising young girl died in front of our eyes. The autopsy confirmed that diphtheritic membrane had occluded all the respiratory passages, including her bronchi, so that nothing we could have done would have restored the patency of her airway.

This experience sobered my outlook as a healer of children. My memory repeatedly brought back the elation of Magali's previous recovery from diphtheria and the gratitude of her parents. These memories were now obscured by an ugly, thick, yellow membrane that covered all the respiratory passages and kept oxygen from reaching her heart and brain. But the most tormenting thought was my ignorance that an attack of diphtheria did not confer natural immunity. Another exposure anytime, anywhere, could result in another bout of diphtheria. Why had this not been mentioned in any of the books or journals I had read? Had no one had a similar terrible experience and reported it to prevent another unnecessary death from diphtheria?

Almost forty years later, my heart is still heavy with grief when I recall this experience. Of all the childhood infectious diseases, diphtheria commands more respect from me than any other. When parents refuse to immunize their children against diphtheria, pertussis and tetanus for fear of seizures, autism, or whatever other reason, I shake my head and wish they knew what I know now.

10

TOXOPLASMOSIS

Toxoplasmosis is a parasitic disease caused by the protozoan *Toxoplasma gondii*, first described by Charles Nicolle, the great French parasitologist, who found it among the gondi, a rodent in Tunisia in 1908. Although initially it was mostly a curiosity, toxoplasmosis was soon found to be prevalent among humans throughout the world and epidemiological studies revealed that the highest incidence occurred among inhabitants in Central America. For example, serological studies showed that in Guatemala more than 90 percent of the population had had toxoplasmosis and in the United States similar studies showed that about 10 to 20 percent of the population had been infected, usually without any or only minimal symptoms.

The fact that such large segments of the population had been infected with *T. gondii* implied that the majority of persons were asymptomatic or only had mild symptoms when toxoplasmosis was acquired. However, when the parasite invades a pregnant woman, it can wreak havoc in the fetus and congenital toxoplasmosis results in a fetus that is severely injured in the brain, eyes and other vital organs. If the affected fetus survives, examination of the eyes will demonstrate the scars of toxoplasmosis in the retina and in the brain there will be calcifications. In patients with HIV, the impaired immune response facilitates the invasion and destruction of tissues by the parasite.

After completing my training in pediatrics in 1967, I worked as a pediatrician at Coco Solo Hospital and then at Gorgas Hospital in the Panama Canal Zone. Across from Gorgas Hospital in Ancon was MARU (Middle America Research Unit), formed by a group of researchers from the U.S. Army, CDC (Communicable Disease Center) and NIH (National Institutes of Health). Among these distinguished experts in the fields of epidemiology, virology, and other tropical diseases, was Colonel Bryce C. Walton.

Walton was a quiet, industrious and most pleasant gentleman whose main interest was toxoplasmosis. I began to attend the weekly conferences at MARU and became excited after hearing about the various investigations reported by the staff. Dr. Karl Johnson was interested in the South American hemorrhagic fevers and one of the members of our hospital had died from Bolivian hemorrhagic fever acquired during a trip to investigate the etiology (a virus) and method of spread (by the urine of the rodent *Calomys callosus*) of the disease. Dr. Pauline Peralta, my sister-in-law, worked as a virologist at MARU and she had also acquired Bolivian hemorrhagic fever but survived and developed a natural immunity to the virus. When another member of the hospital staff came down with Bolivian hemorrhagic fever, she donated her blood and the patient received the separated serum rich in antibodies that saved his life.

Col. Walton showed me his publications and current studies on toxoplasmosis. He explained that toxoplasmosis was also prevalent in the population of Panama. Although the gold standard for testing to see if a person had toxoplasmosis was the Sabin-Feldman methylene blue dye test, this test was complicated and time consuming. Col.

Walton had developed a more accurate and sensitive test, an indirect immunofluorescent antibody test (IFAT), which had been tested and proved to be as good, if not even better, than the Sabin-Feldman method. What he had learned, in addition to the high incidence of toxoplasmosis in Panama, is that a blood titer of antibodies above 1:64 indicated past infection and equal or over 1:1,024 demonstrated an active infection. He also taught me that at times the only clinical evidence of toxoplasmosis was the presence of cervical lymphadenopathy (enlarged neck lymph nodes). Enlarged lymph nodes were common in Panamanian children due to frequent upper respiratory and tonsillopharyngeal infections. However, most of these infections resulted in enlarged nodes in the anterior neck and not in the posterior lymph nodes, which drain mainly the posterior head regions such as the scalp. Infections of the scalp caused by impetigo or scabies would occasionally cause enlargement of the posterior cervical lymph nodes.

Fascinated by what Col. Walton had told me, I began to palpate more carefully the neck in the Panamanian children I saw in the Pediatric Clinic. Anyone I found who had palpably enlarged, non-tender lymph nodes in the back of the neck without impetigo or scabies of the scalp was directed to the laboratory for an indirect immunofluorescent antibody test (IFAT) for toxoplasmosis. The blood was then sent across the street to Col. Walton's laboratory at MARU and the results were ready in about a week. It wasn't long before we had found a dozen or more patients with enlarged neck lymph nodes and elevated titers of more than 1:1,024, indicative of active toxoplasmosis. After many discussions about these patients with Col. Walton, we decided to biopsy some of these lymph nodes and attempt to demonstrate if the parasite was responsible for the swollen lymph nodes.

Lymph nodes act as sentinels and call into action immune cells such as neutrophils, lymphocytes and macrophages, which attack any foreign invader, be it a virus, bacteria, fungus, parasite, or cancer cells, that may result in injury to the host. A careful physical examination includes palpation of the main lymph node groups in the body, such as neck, armpits and groin regions. The presence of enlarged lymph nodes alerts the physician to an infectious or neoplastic (cancerous) process that requires further investigation and treatment.

The surgical removal of a lymph node in the neck was a simple procedure that required only local anesthesia (lidocaine) and a couple of stitches. The biopsy tissue was divided in two or three parts and then carefully placed in vials containing sterile saline and formalin for further studies. The formalin-fixed tissue was sent to pathology for staining and microscopic examination. A portion of the biopsy in sterile saline was sent to bacteriology for cultures and a third portion was sent to Col. Walton's laboratory for research studies. The bacteriology laboratory failed to grow any pathogenic bacteria. The pathologist reported the lymph nodes showed granulomas composed of small groups of epithelioid histiocytes and lymphocytes, reflecting the defense by immune cells against the invading parasites. These histological changes had been previously described in neck lymph nodes and known as *Piringer-Kuchinka* toxoplasmosis lymphadenitis. Numerous attempts to identify the parasite *T. gondii* in the lymph nodes using special stains to make the organism more visible under the microscope also failed to show any direct evidence of the presence of the parasite in the lymph nodes.

Attempts to demonstrate in Col. Walton's laboratory the presence of the toxoplasma parasite in the lymph node tissue using fluorescent antibodies and examining the stained sections under a fluorescent microscope also were unsuccessful. Col. Walton then proceeded to inoculate newborn mice by injecting a portion of the lymph node homogenized and suspended in sterile normal saline. After about ten days, the newborn mice developed swelling of the abdomen due to accumulating peritoneal fluid (ascites). Aspiration of the ascitic fluid revealed under the microscope thousands of living parasites, easily recognized as *T. gondii* due to their characteristic size and shape.

What intrigued me then and continues to intrigue me even now is that we knew that the parasite was present in the lymph nodes but could not see it, at least in its usual morphological appearance. It was "hiding" from us and we were unable to see it. Only the demonstration of the proliferation of the parasite in the newborn mice injected with lymph node material proved that it was already present in the lymph nodes. This was not true of sterile saline injections in newborn mice used as controls.

Although these studies were not published in detail, a letter to *Lancet* reported that we found that these children with toxoplasmosis had more exposure to cats at home or in the neighborhood. The mode of transmission of toxoplasmosis to humans was not known at the time, but cats were suspected as a possible reservoir. Dr. Jack Frenkel, a parasitologist at the Kansas University Medical Center in Kansas City, had been studying this problem for years and he was the most knowledgeable person on toxoplasmosis. The scientific world was thrilled when Frenkel published his admirable studies on the transmission of toxoplasmosis to humans by cats in 1972.

In 1991, I went to work as a pediatric neurologist in the Department of Pediatrics at Kansas University Medical Center. One of the first things I did after my arrival in

Kansas City was to meet with Dr. Frenkel. I went to his laboratory and waited for ten or fifteen minutes until he could take a break from his work. As most dedicated and respected researchers, Frenkel wasted no time and we talked briefly about Col. Walton's work. I told him I had been in Panama and he suddenly recalled that there had been a publication speculating that Dr. Samuel Darling, a pathologist who discovered histoplasmosis while working with William Gorgas during the construction of the Panama Canal, had reported a case of sarcosporidiosis that, from the morphological description and drawings of the parasite, could have been the first case report of human toxoplasmosis. Darling's report was dated 1908, the same year Nicolle and Monceaux found the parasite in Tunisian rodents. It would not be until almost forty years later that the first human case of toxoplasmosis in an adult was published.

Dr. Frenkel got up from his chair and pulled out of the bookshelves a copy (reprint) of the article published in the *Journal of the American Medical Association* (*JAMA*) in 1970. He said, "Here is the article, the author is Enrique Chaves-Carballo." I replied, "That's me."

Chaves-Carballo E: Samuel T. Darling and human sarcosporidiosis or toxoplasmosis in Panama. *Journal of the American Medical Association* (*JAMA*) 1970; 59: 609-612.

Chaves-Carballo E: Toxoplasma antibodies and cats (Letter to the Editor). *Lancet* 1976; 307: 309-310.

Nicolle C, Manceaux L: Sur une infection a corps de Leishman (ou organisms voisins) du gondi. *Comtes Rendus du Academie Sciences* 1908; 147: 763-765.

Darling ST: Sarcosporidiosis, with report of a case in man. *Archives of Internal Medicine* 1909; 4: 150-185.

Piringer-Kuchinka A, Martin I, Thalhammer O: [Superior cervicalnuchal lymphadenitis with small groups of epithelioid cell proliferation.] *Virchows Archiv* 1958; 331: 522-535.

11

YELLOW FEVER

Although I have not seen a single case of yellow fever during my entire medical career, my interest in the medical history of the Panama Canal has familiarized me with this dreadful disease.

Yellow fever was rampant in the South and Margaret Humphreys has written eloquently about it. Yellow fever was responsible, along with malaria, for the failure of the French to complete the interoceanic canal in Panama under their charismatic leader, Ferdinand de Lesseps (builder of the Suez canal), as it decimated the engineering and working forces. It should be understood that at that time, in 1891, yellow fever (as well as malaria) was believed to be caused by *miasmas*, that is, noxious vapors that emanated from nearby swamps due to the decomposition of filth and vegetable matter. At night, folks would entrench themselves behind closed doors and windows from fear of catching what were also known as "swamp fevers."

Two figures have interested me the most while studying the history of yellow fever or *vómito negro* (black vomit), as the Spanish called the disease: Carlos J. Finlay and Clara Maass. Both contributed singularly to the elucidation of the etiology of yellow fever, but in quite different ways. Finlay was a doctor and Maass was a nurse. Finlay was born in Cuba from Scottish and French ancestry. He studied medicine in Philadelphia after he failed to pass the admission examination in Cuba. Aside from his busy clinical practice as an ophthalmologist, Finlay was curious about yellow fever. For years he kept meticulous records on the temperature and humidity in Havana and correlated these with the number of cases of yellow fever in that city. His observations supported the then prevalent miasmatic theory and he presented his findings to the Academy of Sciences in Havana in 1865. The paper was well received and he developed the reputation of a careful and honest scientific investigator.

Finlay was then attached as an observer to the U.S. Army First Yellow Fever Commission, chaired by Stanford Chaillé, a respected pathologist from New Orleans. After examining under the microscope the tissue preparations taken from yellow fever victims and shared by Chaillé, Finlay realized that yellow fever was mainly a hemorrhagic disease caused by damage to the lining of the blood vessels (endothelium) and that the transmission from person to person must be mediated by a vector capable of introducing the virulent agent directly into the circulation. This vector, in Finlay's mind, could only be the mosquito which could penetrate the skin and deposit the instigating agent into the blood using its sharp proboscis. Not only did he then develop his hypothesis of the mosquito-vector transmission of yellow fever in humans, but was also able to identify the specific culprit from many different species found in Havana. The specific mosquito was then called *Stegomyia* and later named *Aedes egypti*. Unfortunately, Finlay was unable to reproduce a single convincing case of yellow fever using religious and military recruits in more than one hundred human inoculation experiments, including himself. But Finlay was totally convinced about the soundness of his hypothesis and presented his findings to the Academy in 1881. The long presentation ended with a complete silence from the audience: no questions, no comments. Everyone thought he was crazy. From then on, Finlay was ridiculed by many of his peers as "the mosquito man." The miasmatic hypothesis had won round one.

Finlay was undaunted. He continued to experiment and talked to anyone who would listen to his ideas about mosquitoes and yellow fever. Fortunately, Finlay was "a kind and lovable man," as Gorgas described him. Gorgas did not believe him either and when Gorgas became Chief Sanitary Officer in Havana, the attack on yellow fever was focused instead on cleaning the city by removing trash and filth. Despite the military-like emphasis on cleaning the city, yellow fever prevailed.

In 1900, Walter Reed was given the task of finding the cause of yellow fever as head of the U.S. Army Fourth Yellow Fever Board. The preceding Third Board had unwittingly found that Giuseppe Sanarelli's claim to have found the cause of yellow fever (which he called *Bacillus icteroides*), was correct. General George Sternberg, then Surgeon General of the U.S. Army and a well-known bacteriologist, became incensed at what he considered an erroneous conclusion by the Board and promptly formed the Fourth Yellow Fever Board composed of, in addition to Reed, contract surgeons James Carroll, Jesse Lazear and Arístides Agramonte. It didn't take long for the newly formed board to refute Sanarelli's claim and to conclude that the offending organism was none other than a contaminating hog-cholera causing bacillus present in the cadavers of yellow fever victims. Rather than wasting time amassing more convincing data against Sanarelli's claim, the members of the board decided to visit Finlay at his home on 100 Aguacate Street in Havana and listen to his ideas. This fateful meeting took place on August 1st, 1900.

Finlay was overwhelmed with emotion and generously shared his copious experimental notes and provided Reed with a porcelain dish containing eggs deposited by the same mosquito Finlay blamed for causing yellow fever. After eight initial unsuccessful inoculations with contaminated mosquitoes (mosquitoes that had been allowed to feed on yellow fever patients) using human volunteers, the members of the board were despondent but kept on trying. Carroll, who did not believe in Finlay's ideas, inoculated himself with "loaded" mosquitoes and within five days came down with an unmistakable and severe case of yellow fever. Another member of the board, Lazear, who did believe Finlay, allowed himself to be bitten by a stray mosquito at Las Animas Hospital, where all yellow fever patients in Havana were admitted, and developed a fatal case of yellow fever. Two additional volunteers were subjected to mosquito inoculations and also developed yellow fever. Although the evidence was meager and subject to further scrutiny, at least one of the cases had been incontrovertible and Reed obtained permission from his superiors to present the preliminary data at the Annual Meeting of the American Association of Public Health in Philadelphia, October 22-26, 1900. Reed's confirmation of Finlay's mosquito vector hypothesis of yellow fever received world acclaim.

Performing additional human experiments under more controlled conditions and using quarantined volunteers, Reed and his board amassed additional evidence that yellow fever was transmitted by mosquitoes, more specifically by Finlay's mosquito. The board also conducted experiments to demonstrate that contaminated objects such as clothing, bedding and other belongings (fomites) from yellow fever victims were incapable of transmitting yellow fever. Reed was careful to acknowledge Finlay's contribution to the elucidation of the mystery of yellow fever. General Leonard Wood convened all the protagonists of this great discovery in a banquet at Delmonico's in Havana to honor Finlay and presented him with a bust to the applause of hundreds present to pay homage to the "mosquito man."

As often happens, the glory of this discovery was insufficient to satisfy all those involved. Animosities developed among Reed, Sternberg, Carroll and Agramonte. These personal squabbles and claims were also elevated to an international level and Cuban physicians and admirers of Finlay reproached the Americans for not giving Finlay due credit. The animosity is still present, more than a century later. Such is human nature.

After Reed's human experiments, Gorgas, Agramonte and Juan Guiteras, a Cuban pathologist educated in the U.S. and professor of pathology at the University of Pennsylvania, decided to try immunizing individuals against yellow fever by giving them a "mild" case of the disease under controlled conditions. Under the direction of Guiteras, an Inoculation Station was created in 1901 at Las Animas Hospital in Havana. Twenty-three volunteers underwent forty-nine inoculation experiments with "loaded" mosquitoes over a period of eight months. It was thought that a mild case of yellow fever could be induced by allowing only a few bites (no more than three) from a single contaminated mosquito. Unfortunately, three of the experimental subjects died as a result: two Spaniards and a twenty-five-year-old American nurse named Clara Louise Maass. All three of the victims had been inoculated with mosquitoes allowed to feed on a young yellow fever patient, Juan Alvarez, who had experienced a severe case but recovered. The "Alvarez mosquitoes" proved beyond any doubt that human immunization against yellow fever using contaminated mosquitoes was not feasible. These deaths resulted in a public outcry and human yellow fever experiments were immediately terminated by the U.S. Army.

Maass' death captured the public's imagination and brought to the forefront the ethics of human experimentation. General Sternberg had admonished against the use of enlisted men for the experiments and permitted volunteers to participate only after their full and informed consent. To Reed's credit, he was the first investigator in the modern era to use a written (both in English and in Spanish) informed consent. The dire consequences of possible deaths weighed heavily on him and, although he was not responsible for the three deaths at Las Animas Hospital, he was appalled when appraised of the results. The reason he was not responsible is that the human experiments at the Inoculation Station were performed under the direction of the Cuban Sanitary Department, presided by Gorgas and not Reed, and the subjects were paid for their participation using Cuban military government and not U.S. Army funds.

Maass was born in New Jersey into a numerous family of nine children as part of the German diaspora that fled Holland to America in search of religious freedom and better opportunities. However, her father was unable to make ends meet and Clara was forced to seek means of supporting her family by working as an unsalaried helper in another family for room and board. She also worked at an orphan asylum feeding, cleaning and caring for orphans ten hours a day for $10 a month, room and board. As the eldest child, she felt responsible for helping her mother pay the bills and decided to become a nurse. Lying about her age, she nevertheless was accepted into nursing school and graduated three years later. Her dedication and lack of aversion to hard work earned her the title of head nurse at the same hospital where she trained. Eager to earn more, she volunteered as a contract nurse during the Spanish-American War and served in military camps in the South and later in the Philippines. She was discharged home after serving nine months because of a severe attack and prolonged convalescence due to dengue.

Typhoid fever was the major killer of American soldiers during the Spanish-American War. For every battle casualty, seven men died of infectious diseases. More men died from bacilli than from bullets. Several exhaustive investigations revealed the appalling lack of hygiene at military camps. Although initially Sternberg agreed with his officers that there was no place for female nurses in the camps and hospitals of the U.S. Army, he soon realized that female nurses not only were better trained than their male counterparts in the application and understanding of sanitary measures, but also provided wounded and sick soldiers with the soothing and compassionate touch only females were capable of giving. As a result, Sternberg changed his position and allowed the recruitment of female nurses and the U.S. Army Nurse Corps was created in 1901. More than fifty thousand trained female nurses were hired by the U.S. Army based on their qualifications of professional ability, good character and health. Their salary was $30 a month, laundry of their uniforms and one daily ration.

When American nurses were needed in Cuba, Clara volunteered and Gorgas, who was well aware of her nursing skills, answered her with a terse telegram "Come at once." This she did and when she found out about the yellow fever vaccinations at Las Animas Hospital, she eagerly volunteered. Despite her repeated exposure to yellow fever patients in Santiago, Cuba, during the

Spanish-American War, Maass was not immune to yellow fever and wished to acquire the disease under controlled conditions. Furthermore, each volunteer was paid $100 U.S. gold and an additional $100 U.S gold if he or she came down with an attack of experimental yellow fever. On five different occasions, Maass was inoculated with "loaded" mosquitoes but she did not develop yellow fever. On August 14, 1901, she submitted herself for the sixth time. However, this time she became gravely ill, suffered a particularly virulent attack and died ten days later.

When Maass came down with yellow fever, she sent a poignant letter to her mother:

> *Goodbye, Mother,*
> *Don't worry. God will take care of me in the yellow*
> *fever hospital the same as if I were at home.*
> *I will send you nearly all I earn, so be good to*
> *yourself and the two little ones.*
> *You know I am the man of the family, but do pray*
> *for me.*

Gorgas informed her family of Clara's death in another terse telegram on August 24, 1901:

> *Miss Maas[s] died twenty fourth six thirty pm.*

Clara was secretly engaged to be married to a businessman from New York and she had asked her sister, Sophia, who also was a nurse, to come to Cuba and relieve Clara of her nursing duties. Sophia arrived in Cuba not knowing of the death of her sister until she landed in Havana.

The members of the U.S. Army Fourth Yellow Fever Board had pledged to inoculate themselves first before using other volunteers. Both Carroll and Lazear did but paid a price: Carroll never completely recovered from cardiac complications and Lazear gave his life. It is not clear why Reed did not submit himself to mosquito inoculations. At age forty-three, he did confess fear of not surviving an attack of experimental yellow fever. His untimely death from appendicitis scarcely two years after the epochal discovery may have spared him considerable criticism for the dangerous human experiments in Cuba. For reasons that remain unclear, Gorgas and Guiteras, who supervised the failed immunization studies at Las Animas Hospital, were not incriminated or blamed for Clara Maass' death. The wrath of the newspapers appeared to be directed more to the U.S. Army. A reporter in the *New Jersey Evening News*, quoted Clara's mother as saying, "To me, from all I know, my daughter's death was nothing short of murder."

The ethics of human experimentation have been the subject of many discussions. Jenner's inoculation of a child with the cowpox virus and Pasteur's vaccination of a human subject with the rabies vaccine centuries back, although resulting in incalculable benefits to humanity, probably would not have been approved by any Institutional Review Board (IRB) today. The Nuremberg trials of Nazi atrocities and the Helsinki declaration signaled a new era of ethical guidelines for human experimentation. One of the most important ethical principles was stated in article 5 of the Helsinki Declaration (article 6 in the 2008 revision) indicating clearly that in medical research involving humans, the well being of the individual research subject should take precedence over the interests of science and society. No longer could human experimentation be justified as in the past because possible harm to the human subject was overridden by results that could benefit mankind. This was no longer acceptable and the rights of the individual superseded any considerations to benefit other humans.

Whatever Clara Maass' motives for volunteering may have been—altruism, desire to become immune or monetary compensation—responsibility for her death falls squarely on the shoulders of those who supervised the human experiments. In this sense, Gorgas and Guiteras still owe us an explanation. Rodríguez-Expósito, one of the latter's biographers, stated that Guiteras was so affected by Maass' death that he never talked about it again and when he became Chief Sanitary Officer in Cuba, he rejected outright mass childhood vaccination as being too dangerous for public health purposes.

Clara Maass was honored by Cuba on the twenty-fifth anniversary following her death by emitting a stamp showing her profile and a picture of Las Animas Hospital. A bronze plaque was placed on the ward where she died but this was removed later by the Fidel Castro regime. The U.S. Postal Service issued a stamp in her honor on the fiftieth anniversary of her sacrifice. Perhaps the most lasting recognition is the naming of the hospital where she trained and worked as the Clara Maass Medical Center, now located in Belleville, New Jersey. A small museum in the hospital functions as a repository for her letters, photographs and other memorabilia.

The identification of *Aedes egypti* as the mosquito vector of yellow fever dispelled all previous ideas that miasmas caused yellow fever and malaria. Gorgas' application of the derived mosquito control measures resulted in the eradication of yellow fever in Havana for the first time in one hundred and fifty years. This knowledge also made possible the successful completion of the Panama Canal by the Americans in 1914.

Chaves-Carballo E: Carlos Finlay and yellow fever: Triumph over adversity. *Military Medicine* 2005; 170: 881-5.

Chaves-Carballo E: Clara Maass, yellow fever and human experimentation. (Accepted for publication in *Military Medicine*.)

12

GERM OF LAZINESS

The World Health Organization (WHO) estimates that seven hundred forty million people worldwide are infested with hookworm. This ailment belongs to the group now denoted as soil-transmitted diseases. The new name does not improve the lack of public health and hygienic measures mainly responsible for the perpetuation and propagation of hookworm among the poor and developing countries in the world.

Hookworm is an intestinal parasite found in fecally-contaminated soil. The dormant larvae, under the right conditions, emerge and penetrate the skin of barefoot humans. From there the parasite enters the venous circulation to the lungs, reaches the alveoli (pulmonary air sacs) and is then coughed and swallowed to reach a final destination, the small intestine. The parasite attaches itself to the intestinal wall by using the specialized hooks around its oral opening and causes microscopic bleeding. Intestinal infestation by a few hundred of these worms results in chronic anemia and general lassitude.

In 1902, Charles Wardell Stiles became convinced that the lack of drive and ambition in the South could be explained by the prevalence of hookworm, which he called "the germ of laziness." Using his rhetoric and pulpit-acquired communication skills, Stiles was able to convince the Rockefeller Foundation to embark on a hookworm eradication campaign in the South. The purported success of this public health initiative led the Foundation to launch a worldwide hookworm eradication campaign, in keeping with its ambitious goals to promote "the well-being of mankind throughout the world."

The hookworm parasite has evolved into two similar but morphologically distinct species: the "old world" *Ancylostoma duodenale* and the "new world" *Necator americanus*. Samuel T. Darling, the great American pathologist/parasitologist, chose an analysis of hookworm in different populations as the topic for his presidential address to the annual meeting of the American Society of Tropical Medicine in 1925: "Comparative helminthology as an aid in the solution of ethnological problems." Unfortunately, Darling was unable to deliver this paper, as he died in an automobile accident near Beirut only a few months before the meeting.

The Rockefeller emissaries (sanitary inspectors) were equipped with a Bausch & Lomb collapsible microscope designed to fit in a saddlebag, a supply of medicines, literature, photographs, charts and lantern slides for educational purposes. The success of Rockefeller's initial five year eradication plan in the South was measured by the fact that over one million stool examinations and half a million people were treated for hookworm. The recipients of the international campaign included developing countries in Latin America and in the Far East such as Puerto Rico, Philippines, Malaya and Panama.

When Lewis Hackett arrived in Panama in 1914 to head the Rockefeller intent to eradicate hookworm and other intestinal parasites there, he kept on his desk a glass jar containing two thousand hookworms removed from a ten-year-old child whose anemic blood and pallor were reflected in a hemoglobin value of only 10 percent of the "normal richness and color." Population studies in Panama showed that 69 percent of the children harbored intestinal parasites and that of these, one in ten was infested with at least two or more different parasites. A simple procedure, wearing shoes, helped to break the evolving life cycle of hookworm, while a more complex and expensive public health program of constructing latrines and sewer systems, helped to reduce the "germ of laziness".

Ettling J: *The Germ of Laziness. Rockefeller Philanthropy and Public Health in the New South.* Cambridge, MA: Harvard University Press, 1981.

13

TUBERCULOSIS VACCINE

Protection against tuberculosis is commonly attempted in developing countries by inoculation of children with an attenuated live strain of mycobacteria known as *Bacille Calmette-Guérin* or, more simply, BCG.

Albert Calmette and Camille Guérin, French investigators at the Pasteur Institute, developed BCG by taking a strain of bovine tuberculosis, *Mycobacterium bovis*, and reducing its virulence after two hundred and thirty passages over a thirteen year period in artificial media. BCG was first tested in humans in 1927 and found to be about 80 percent effective in protecting against tuberculosis for at least five years. As a result, most countries use BCG vaccination programs to protect populations from tuberculosis. However, early studies in the United States found BCG to be much less efficacious and tuberculosis surveillance was implemented instead with the Mantoux (tuberculin) test. A positive Mantoux test indicates the subject has recently been exposed to tuberculosis and further treatment determined with chest x-rays and testing of all possible contacts.

When American health authorities arrived in Panama in preparation for the construction of the Panama Canal in the early 1900s, pneumonia and tuberculosis were found to be the leading causes of death. The canal laborers came mainly from Jamaica and Barbados and were housed in crowded quarters with poor ventilation and deficient nutrition. Other studies suggest that the young labor force had decreased resistance to pneumococcal (pneumonia microbe) infections.

When I arrived in Panama as an intern at Gorgas Hospital in 1963, every patient admitted had a mandatory chest x-ray done before arriving to the ward. I did not understand the reason for this policy until the radiologist started calling back on a regular basis reporting that many of the patients I admitted had pulmonary tuberculosis. Before the clinical availability of x-rays (then called *skiagraphs*), physicians relied mainly on their clinical abilities to detect lung lesions by using auscultation and percussion. As in any human endeavor, practice makes perfect and these astute clinicians were able to diagnose pneumonia and tuberculosis by hearing abnormal breath sounds such as râles, rhonchi, dullness to percussion and ventriloquy (the distortion of sounds when the patient speaks as detected with the stethoscope). Unfortunately, such clinical skills have been long lost and no longer learned by medical students and residents since x-rays, computerized tomography (CT) and magnetic resonance imaging (MRI) are now more accurate and accessible. Today, the stethoscope is proudly displayed around the neck by younger physicians but they seldom know how to use it well, while in those days it was discretely protected inside the coat pocket as befitted one of our most prized possessions.

Before the year of rotating internship in Panama was completed, I had converted from negative to positive when tested with the Mantoux test for tuberculosis. However, chest x-rays done yearly since have been negative for tuberculosis, except for detection of a possible Ghon complex (a calcified lymph node in the lungs). When a person first encounters tuberculosis bacilli entering the respiratory tract and lungs, defenses immediately come to the aid and surround the invaders with defending cells such as lymphocytes and macrophages located in a lymph node that may then become calcified. This prison from which the tuberculosis bacilli cannot escape and cause more damage is known as a Ghon complex. The presence of the bacilli, even if these have died, results in a Mantoux positive reaction. A positive Mantoux test remains so for years, if not for life. Because a positive test sets off an alarm of public health proportions in the United States, at times it is difficult to explain why I refuse to be tested for tuberculosis in this manner. The last time I had a Mantoux test many years ago, the redness and induration produced in my forearm measured over ten centimeters (about four inches) and was quite painful.

I returned to Panama after completing my training as a pediatrician in 1967. BCG immunization was routinely given at the time to Panamanian children in our hospital. Between August 1968 and December 1969, 1,295 children were given BCG in the Canal Zone. Each child had to have a negative Mantoux test prior to vaccination and BCG was injected intradermally (not subcutaneously) in the left deltoid region. Although intradermal injection was not easy, nursing personnel became quite adept in the proper administration of BCG.

Shortly after the vaccination program began in that year, we began to see children who had developed enlargement of a left axillary (armpit) lymph node as a result of the reaction to BCG. This was neither unusual nor unexpected. However, we found children who not only had developed an enlarged lymph node, but the node suppurated (drained pus) and despite all our efforts to suppress this with antibiotics and topical ointments, continued to drain for days and weeks.

We kept close track of the numbers. Of 1,295 children vaccinated with BCG, twenty-five (or 1.9 percent) developed lymph node enlargement. Of these, about half or twelve cases, went on to drain pus externally anywhere from one to eleven months after vaccination. Non-suppurative BCGitis, as we decided to call this reaction, regressed spontaneously within a few weeks or months. Suppurating BCGitis tended to heal more slowly and required up to eight months for spontaneous cicatrization (scarring) and closure. Specific antituberculous treatment was given to two of the children in the form of isoniazid (INH) but this did not accelerate healing. The remaining cases of suppurating BCGitis were treated surgically and this was followed by prompt healing and cessation of pus drainage. Microscopic examination of the excised lymph nodes showed exactly the same lesions as seen in tuberculosis, with granulomas, caseation necrosis and typical Langerhans giant cells.

Since BCG was introduced nearly a century ago, adverse reactions have been described (including deaths) in children given BCG. Enlargement of armpit lymph nodes may result from faulty injection techniques or, more commonly, from vaccine not sufficiently attenuated, so that the live *Mycobacterium bovis* is more aggressive and destroys more tissue. Detailed examination of the provenance of the BCG vaccine lots used in the Canal Zone showed that eight of the cases of BCGitis had been given vaccine from Lot #11 and four from Lot #13. The other cases received BCG from six other scattered lots. As soon as the responsible lots were identified, these were removed and BCG from then on was purchased from a different supplier. As far as I am aware, these were the only examples of BCGitis seen in the Canal Zone for decades afterwards.

Some of the enlarged and draining lymph nodes were quite large, resembling a small lemon. By now I had acquired a versatile and inexpensive Startech® camera developed by Kodak® mainly for dental photography. The camera had a string of metal beads with two colored beads to mark the correct distance to place the object or subject and two interchangeable lenses for each close distance. I believe this camera cost about $25 at the time. I took hundreds of slides of interesting tropical lesions using Kodak Ektachrome® 35-mm color film and had these developed at the Panafoto store in Panama City. My vast collection of interesting slides helped me to give each year two one-hour lectures on tropical pediatrics to students and residents, showing them examples of unusual and interesting cases they otherwise would not have seen. As often said, "a picture is worth a thousand words."

Chaves-Carballo E: Regional lymphadenitis following BCG vaccination (BCGitis). *Clinical Pediatrics* 1972; 11: 693-697.

14

MIGHTY MITES

Skin lesions are among the most common problems seen in the tropics. The abundance of insects, heat and humidity, as well as outdoor activities, conspire together to breach the integrity of the skin. Children, particularly, are prone to abrasions, cuts and scrapes, which quickly become infected. These skin infections are known as *impetigo* and constituted a good portion of the pediatric patients brought to our clinics in Panama.

What appeared unusual was that many of the children had impetigo in areas not typically exposed to sunlight or insects, as in the creases of the arms and legs and in the skin folds interdigitally (between the fingers). By the time these children were seen in the clinic, the skin lesions were covered with pus or crusted material. Another unusual aspect of the skin lesions was intense itching, which resulted in vigorous scratching and additional injury to the skin and spread of the infection. Resorting to my trusted clinical tools—a magnifying glass and a Swiss Army pocket knife—I was determined to find out what was causing these intensely pruritic lesions. After several scrapings and examining these under a microscope, an appendage appeared which suggested a very small arthropod or mite might be the culprit. More vigorous and deeper digging showed the unmistakable appearance of *Sarcoptes scabiei*. This "mighty mite" causes mange in animals but can adapt easily to humans and can be transmitted by close contact between infested individuals. The intense itching and typical distribution of scabies became easily recognized and soon the yearly hospital supply of a scabicidal medication was exhausted in the first few months due to its increased demand in the clinic.

The scabies parasite is almost invisible to the naked eye and measures less than half-a-millimeter in diameter, with four pairs of short legs, and resembles the shape of a turtle. The female burrows into the skin, where she deposits eggs that later hatch into larvae and mature into adult mites. The intense itching, which was thought to be caused by the burrowing, may be also due to some immune response by the host. The skin lesions easily become infected with bacteria and the infected lesions are known as impetigo.

One of the many medical curiosities encountered in Panama was a high incidence of acute glomerulonephritis in children. Acute glomerulonephritis is an inflammation of the kidney that damages the filtrating units (glomeruli) where impurities in the blood are filtered out into the urine. This results also in the presence of hematuria (blood in the urine), easily detected in microscopic analysis of urine. Acute glomerulonephritis is caused by streptococcal infections. Certain streptococci may produce specific toxins that damage the kidneys, and these are called nephritogenic strains.

Many cultures of impetiginous lesions in our children with scabies consistently showed the presence of both streptococcal and staphylococcal bacteria (*Streptococcus pyogenes* and *Staphylococcus aureus*). Studies in Trinidad had demonstrated that acute glomerulonephritis could be caused by specific strains of streptococci that were nephritogenic, that is, could damage the kidney. The investigator who first reported this was Elizabeth Potter in Chicago. After corresponding with

Potter, she expressed interest in investigating the relationship between scabies and acute glomerulonephritis in Panama. The methodology was fairly simple. Impetigo lesions were cultured in our laboratory and the streptococci suspended in sterile broth. The broth was then impregnated on sterile filter paper and dried in an incubator at 37° C. The filter paper was then covered with aluminum foil, folded and sent in an envelope by airmail to Chicago. This simple method devised by Potter worked well and no samples were lost. In her laboratory, Potter isolated the Panamanian streptococcal strains and compared these with those she had found in Trinidad. Most of the strains from Panama were new strains and were given new M-type numbers to distinguish them from older strains. Potter published these findings in several articles and established that acute glomerulonephritis was commonly caused by impetigo lesions produced by scabies and colonized by nephritogenic strains of streptococci in Panama. Damage to the kidneys, therefore, could be traced back all the way to infected scabetic lesions. Once again, the complexity of parasitic lesions in the tropics never ceased to amaze me.

Potter EV, Siegel AC, Simon NM, et al: Streptococcal infections and epidemic glomerulonephritis in South Trinidad. *Journal of Pediatrics* 1968; 72: 871-84.

15

NECK MAGGOTS

The most common causes of cervical lymphadenopathy (enlargement of the neck lymph nodes) in Panamanian children were scalp or skin infections caused by bacteria (streptococcus and staphylococcus) and known as impetigo. Another less common etiology was toxoplasmosis, a parasitic infection transmitted by cats. A rather unusual but also well-known cause for nodular swelling in the neck was *myasis*.

Myasis is the name given to the invasion of skin or mucous membranes in humans by the larvae of the botfly, also known as *Dermatobia hominis*. The botfly deposits her eggs on the skin of a warm-blooded animal such as cattle. As the eggs develop into larvae, the latter burrow under the skin and grow by absorbing nutrients from the surrounding tissue. The larvae reach a considerable size (about half-inch in length) and appear to live comfortably in these circumstances. Because of their ability to clean or debride necrotic or dead tissue, dipterous (insects with one pair of functional wings) larvae (maggots) have been used effectively in the past to clean nasty wounds. This practice has more recently been revived with limited use.

Among the many children seen in the hospital clinic with enlarged neck nodes, there were some not explained by infection or toxoplasmosis after careful inspection and palpation of the nodes and antibody studies in blood. The lesions were not painful, unattached to surrounding tissue and not a reason for complaints by the patients. One day, using my pocket magnifying glass and cleaning as much as possible with alcohol swabs the skin over a node, I saw something wiggle inside through a small, almost imperceptible opening. What appeared to be an optical illusion at first, with some patience and perspicacity, became a source of interest. Yes! There was something moving under the skin. Using local anesthesia and sterile scissors, a small cut showed the presence of a wiggling larva or maggot, which was easily extracted with fine forceps and placed in a formalin bottle. Usually there would be more than one of these but not more than two or three, which were similarly removed.

Although telling mothers that there were living maggots under the skin of the neck in her child may sound repulsive, most Panamanians were familiar with this occurring in cattle and known locally as *tórsalo*. They were usually grateful that we had removed these parasites from their children. The fly responsible for myasis belongs to the genus *Tabanidae*, also known in Spanish as *tábanos*. The flies are persistent, as most flies are, and a nagging child like myself used to be called by that name many years ago.

While doing research for a book on American medicine in Panama during the construction of the Panama Canal, I found several unusual examples of myasis reported in the *Proceedings of the Canal Zone Medical Association*. Three separate reports documented rather revolting instances of myasis. One was the almost complete covering by thousands of long, black larvae identified as *Hermetia illucens* or "black-soldier fly" on a cadaver found in the jungle several weeks later after an apparent suicide. The second case was that of a twenty-three-year-old man who had myasis of the scrotum. The third and most grotesque case was that of a Panamanian admitted to the hospital because of exquisite tenderness and swelling of one side of his face and a foul, serosanguineous discharge from his left nostril. Nasal irrigations with one-half percent carbolic acid yielded two days later a larva three-quarters of an inch long. After cocainization of the mucous membrane and plugging the nostril with cotton soaked in chloroform, a total of seventy-one worms was recovered and identified as *Chrysomia marcellaria*. Among the comments that followed this case presentation, one of the doctors reported that he had seen many of these cases and the maximum number of worms he had obtained was two-hundred fifty from one patient! The meetings of the Canal Zone Medical Association were usually accompanied by food from the hospital cafeteria but I doubt that many had a hearty appetite after this presentation.

Bishop W.A.: Two types of skin myasis. *Proceedings of the Isthmian Canal Zone Medical Association* 1915; VII (Part 2): 87-93.

16

MOON CHILDREN

Albinism is one of the four hereditary diseases studied by Sir Archibald Garrod in the Eighteenth Century (the others were alkaptonuria, cystinuria and pentosuria) and to which he gave the name of *inborn errors of metabolism*. Garrod consolidated his ideas and investigations in his Croonian lectures given in 1908 and later published in the English medical journal *Lancet*.

Albinism, Garrod explained, is caused by absence of pigment and this is inherited as an autosomal recessive characteristic. Those who have this hereditary defect are known as albinos. Garrod's contributions included co-authorship of the first pediatric textbook addressing pediatric neurology, *Diseases of Children*, published in 1913 and co-authored by Fred Batten and Hugh Thursfield. Garrod's seminal contributions on the concepts of chemical individuality and inborn errors of metabolism were not appreciated (reminiscent of Mendel's seminal contributions in genetics two decades earlier) until many years later.

The Kuna Indians of Panama at one time had the highest incidence of albinism in the world. They called their albino children the *moon children* and, although they considered them to be special, separated these from the rest of the village in a remote hut where they received food, clothing and daily care. The purpose of such quarantine methods is not clear, but may have been based on the belief that albinism could be contagious and, therefore, the need to isolate those affected. In the Kuna mythology, moon children defended the moon from devouring dragons.

The Kuna Indians are a fiercely independent, highly intelligent and enterprising group of native Americans. Their society is a matriarchal one, so that when a daughter marries, her husband goes to work for her father and adopts her last name. It is the woman who keeps the earnings from the sale of coconuts and she wears the wealth as gold ornaments: a gold ring on her nose, gold arm bracelets and gold coins in necklaces. Kuna women are industrious and will sew with great skill colorful renditions of animals, birds and fish, as well as figures from books or magazines, using panels of cloth superimposed on each other in a process called *reverse appliqué*. Sewing during most of the daylight hours and using tiny stitches (some less than 1 mm in length) for about a week, the final product called a *mola*, is ready for sale to tourists and interior decorators. The highly valued molas of yesteryear, each one of which was a unique creation by one of these talented women, have since given way to mass-produced ones using sewing machines and intense colors, such as yellows and greens, instead of the muted reds and oranges that at one time identified the best molas. The price of molas has always been reasonable, taking into account the number of hours spent in making them. For many years they were sold for $5, then $10, and now $20. However, the same mola, once framed artistically and exhibited in a New York boutique, will demand several hundred dollars. Mola collection can be a time- and money-consuming hobby. A hospital director in Panama once showed me a trunkful with about five hundred molas from his personal collection.

The Canal Zone Isthmian Anthropological Society came up with the idea of producing a small monograph on molas for sale to tourists as a means to raise funds for our activities. The result was a forty-six page booklet with black-and-white illustrations which sold for $1. This became a popular item for tourists and sold well for a number of years until more colorful and elaborate books on molas appeared on the market.

The Kunas, as mentioned, have their own language and a governing hierarchy. Although they are considered part of the Republic of Panama, they obey their own rules and major decisions are made by a council of elders, led by their chief or *cacique*. The Kunas lived at one time near the Bayano River in the mainland but moved to the San Blas Islands on the Caribbean away from mosquitoes and other disease-carrying insects. The San Blas archipelago consists of hundreds of tiny islands rising only a few feet above the water level. The region inhabited by the Kunas is known as the *comarca* (reservation) of San Blas and the seat of their government is in the larger island of Matapali.

As many other indigenous peoples, Kunas have their own arsenal of natural remedies used to treat their ailments and the *shaman* is the healer who uses herbs and incantations to cure patients. Nevertheless, the parents brought their sick children to our hospital when their traditional remedies failed to give the desired results. Taking a medical history from Jamaicans, Panamanians or other ethnic groups could be a difficult task—but not so with Kunas. Their answers were usually precise and accurate, which to my way of thinking, demonstrated their great intellect.

Because of the lack of pigment in the retina, albinos have poor vision and develop abnormal eye movements called *pendular nystagmus*. This type of nystagmus, where the eyes move to-and-fro in equal excursions (and hence the name pendular) differs from nystagmus related to vestibular or cerebellar disorders, in which the movements consist of a quick and then followed by a slower horizontal movement of the eye. This same type of nystagmus also occurs when we are looking out the window from a moving vehicle or train. Pendular nystagmus, however, indicates congenital blindness or loss of vision that begins early in life.

The unanswered question in my mind, as a pediatrician, was: how early in life does pendular nystagmus develop in albino children? The medical literature I searched seemed to be silent on this. Was it right after birth, one or two days later, or was it after weeks or months? No one that I asked knew the answer. The opportunity came to find out when a Kuna baby was born in our hospital. With the mother's permission, the infant was kept in our newborn nursery and everyday I went to check the eyes for nystagmus. Pendular nystagmus was not present at birth nor in the next few days. It was only about two weeks later when the baby started to look and follow faces that pendular nystagmus clearly developed. This made a lot of sense. Pendular nystagmus developed when the infant acquired useful vision that allowed him or her to identify the mother's face. But this was only one observation in one albino baby and these findings could not be generalized to all albino infants. Unfortunately, this was the only albino born in our hospital during the four years I was there and no firm conclusions could be made on the basis of a single case.

Chaves E, Argenmuller L: *About Molas*. 1969, 46 pp.

Garrod AE: Inborn errors of metabolism. The Croonian lectures delivered before the Royal College of Physicians of London. *Lancet* 1908; II: 1-7, 73-9, 142-8, 214-20.

17

HEAD LICE

Life in the tropics is complicated by a constant struggle between insects and humans. The most admirable adaptation is that of the malaria mosquito vector, *Anopheles albimanus*, which serves as an obligatory host for the malaria parasite to complete its complicated life cycle. Malaria, yellow fever and dengue are only a few of the serious human afflictions mediated by insects in tropical lands. Heat and humidity facilitate the proliferation of many species of insects, from chiggers to mites to flies to spiders to scorpions, all of which become pests, some even poisonous, to torment the otherwise paradisiac existence of those who prefer to sleep in a hammock rather than on an expensive firm mattress.

Before the advent of pesticides such as D.D.T. and chlordane, treatment of head lice consisted of physical removal of the parasite and its eggs (nits) with a fine-tooth comb. The long-time association of lice with humans has been perpetuated in the adaptation in our lexicon of "lousy," "nit-picking," and, of course, "a fine-tooth comb." The fine-tooth comb was made of *carey* from the conch of the turtle. Combing hair to detect and remove lice and nits was never pleasant, since hair shafts often were pulled out from the scalp altogether during this maneuver. In Panama, our hospital would run out of a whole year's supply of medication for treatment of head lice (also known as pediculosis), during the first few months of the year.

Head lice are transmitted directly among humans by close head-to-head contact. The infestation causes intense itching due to the penetration of the scalp by the insect's proboscis (feeding tube) and excretion of irritating saliva near the feeding site. A couple of head shampoos with the lice medication would eradicate most of the insects and eggs.

I had long forgotten about head lice until a resurgence among school children in the U.S. reminded us that the pest was still with us. On one of my return trips to Costa Rica, I found my mother scratching her head vigorously. When I examined her scalp, there they were: both lice and nits in abundance! She claimed she probably acquired the infestation at the city market, but who knows. A quick trip to the local pharmacy and two applications of a medicated shampoo provided lasting relief.

Although I myself had not experienced head lice, fleas were daily (or should I say nightly) companions. The telltale sign of precisely placed and spaced red lesions on my abdomen indicated the next morning that it had been a good feeding excursion for the fleas. Trying to kill the fleas by crushing them between our thumbnails was nothing more than an exercise in futility. The advent of D.D.T. and later, chlordane, changed all that. The powder effectively eradicated fleas from our lives. Such a blessing, of course, could not last long and after Rachel Carson's *Silent Spring*, one after another pesticide was banned because of harm to the environment. The insects won the battle and fleas continue to pester humans all over the world.

A lesser known ectoparasite but well-known to me during my childhood was the *nigua* or tungiasis, caused by the smallest known flea, *Tunga penetrans*. Less than one mm in size, the female borrows through the skin between the toes near the toenail and causes a small, red blister which is intensely pruritic (itchy). As the female lays her eggs, the blister enlarges and can become infected to produce a small periungual abscess. The only remedy in those days was to extirpate the *nigua* with a clean needle followed by an application of alcohol. The procedure was painful and not a favorite of mine.

Co-existence with insects in the tropics is a fact of life. Rather than become exasperated by the constant intrusion in our lives by these tiny enemies, I prefer to study and admire their adaptability and marvel at their ability to extract from humans whatever they need to survive. In that sense, insects appear to be at the top of the food chain, since they partake of our blood and skin while they do not appear to offer us in turn any benefit. I call this the "tropical democracy" because everyone, be it humans or insects, survives by adapting to each other.

18

MALARIA

Malaria remains one of the leading causes of death among children in the world. It is estimated that more than one million children under the age of five years die yearly from cerebral malaria, mainly in the sub-Saharan continent. The malaria parasite invades the brain and produces swelling (cerebral edema) and death.

Despite the devastation it causes, I have long admired the malaria parasite and studied meticulously its prodigious ability to survive along with its complex life cycle. The name "malaria" was given to the disease many centuries ago when "bad airs" or *miasmas* that arose from decomposition of filth and vegetable matter in swamps near human habitats were blamed for the disease. Even in tropical regions where heat and humidity demanded ventilation, the fear of miasmatic vapors made inhabitants close all doors and windows to protect themselves from noxious vapors that caused "swamp fever", "Chagres fever", "tertian and quartan fevers" (depending on the number of days between attacks of fever and chills), recurrent fever, or, in its deadliest form caused by *Plasmodium falciparum* and previously known as "malignant fever."

Alphonse Laveran (1845-1922), a French parasitologist, saw for the first time under the microscope the parasite in the blood of patients with malaria in Algeria. Ronald Ross (1857-1932), a British physician, while in

Islamabad, India, was able to decipher the complex life cycle of the malaria parasite in the mosquito. Quinine, extracted from the cinchona bark, was known by the indigenous people of South America to cure fevers. A Jesuit priest used this medicinal extract to cure the Marquise de Cinchon from her malarial fever. Quinine remained the "specific" for treatment of malaria for over four centuries until, during the Vietnam War, malaria was found to be resistant to treatment with chloroquine (a safer derivative of quinine) near the Cambodian border. American soldiers involved in the conflict suffered from recurrent attacks of malaria due to drug-resistant malaria. Soon thereafter, drug-resistant malaria also was reported from Colombia and other South American countries.

The successful completion of the Panama Canal by the Americans in 1914 was made possible by the investment in sanitation measures instituted by Col. William Gorgas, who eradicated yellow fever and controlled malaria in Panama. The two diseases had been responsible for the unsuccessful attempt by the French in constructing an interoceanic route in Panama in 1881. Although malaria was not completely eradicated by the Americans in Panama, a comfortable truce between man and the parasite was established in the early Twentieth Century.

The emergence of drug-resistant malaria was of much concern to both American and Panamanian health authorities. Active surveillance had failed, however, to indicate any drug-resistant cases of malaria in the region until almost seventy years later.

In October 1969, a number of children with malaria were admitted to Coco Solo Hospital, on the Atlantic side of the Canal Zone. After treatment with amodiaquine (a derivative of quinine), the children appeared to be cured and were sent home with no evidence of malaria parasites on examination of their blood. However, within two or three weeks, the same children returned with chills and fever. A logical explanation was that they had returned home, to the same environment where mosquitoes laden with malaria parasites bit them again and the whole cycle was repeated. The only complete solution to the problem was to eradicate the mosquitoes in the area where they lived, an almost impossible task. But what if the recurrent chills and fever were due to drug-resistant malaria? This was an important question not to be dismissed lightly because of the strategic and commercial importance of the Panama Canal.

Obtaining permission to admit the children to the hospital and keeping them there for prolonged intervals was not difficult. Parents were happy to know that their children would be staying in an air-conditioned ward, eating wholesome American food, playing with toys and taken care of by American doctors and nurses whom they admired and respected. Parents and other family members could visit them anytime they wished. This was the only way I could think of to prove the existence of drug-resistant malaria: not allowing the children to return to their homes, where the risk of acquiring malaria again was high.

Between October 31 and November 22, 1969, three children ages 4, 7 and 10 years, were admitted to Coco Solo Hospital and kept there from 44 to 61 days. Blood was obtained daily by finger-pricks and the blood smears examined for malaria parasites. All the children appeared to be initially cured from malaria and the parasites disappeared from their blood following treatment with amodiaquine. However, nine to nineteen days later, chills and fever returned and the blood smears now showed malaria parasites. A second or even third round of treatment with amodiaquine did not completely eradicate the parasites, proving for the first time the presence of drug-resistant malaria in Panama. However, treatment with quinine was effective and malaria did not recur. Confident of my findings and aware of the importance of this discovery, the results were presented to a military medical meeting where these were received with interest. I then went to the authorities at the Gorgas Memorial Laboratory in Panama City to report and alert them of the results. However, they told me I was wrong and that their careful surveillance all over the country showed no evidence of drug-resistant malaria in Panama. I knew I was right and that they were wrong, but hoped they would pay attention and redouble their efforts before it was too late. Within three years, the malaria experts published their own findings in the *American Journal of Tropical Medicine & Hygiene* and took all the credit for the discovery.

The experience taught me a valuable lesson. I learned that not all medical investigators are honest and that prejudices and jealousies sometimes cloud their scientific judgment. I also learned that satisfaction comes from the results of our work and not from what others think about it. My satisfaction was greater knowing that these children did not have to continue suffering from recurrent attacks of malignant fever.

Chaves Carballo E: Los niños de Escobal, el Hospital Coco Solo y la malaria resistente en Panamá [The children of Escobal, Coco Solo Hospital and drug-resistant malaria in Panama]. *Revista Cultural de Panamá La Lotería* 2010; No. 491 (July-August): 64-71.

Young MD, Johnson CM: Plasmodium falciparum malaria in Panama resistant to 4-aminoquinoline drugs. *American Journal of Tropical Medicine & Hygiene* 1972; 21: 13-7.

III

SICK BRAINS

19

MIGRAINE

The attacks of migraine came with uncanny regularity. Every few months my mother experienced attacks of severe headaches and vomiting and the diagnosis of *jaquecas* or migraine was recognized and accepted by everyone. Her remedies consisted of *espíritu de azahar* (essence of orange blossoms), which had a calming effect and lemon juice as an astringent to settle down her stomach. When more severe, she would experience shaking chills that rocked the bed back and forth. Salicylate solution and alcohol applications were then added to the limited pharmacopeia at our disposal.

On one occasion, the attack of migraine was so severe that a call was made for Dr. Nilo Villalobos to come to see her. Dr. Villalobos was a tall, quiet man who had studied medicine in Belgium and had the innate ability to inspire trust and confidence in his patients, particularly in my mother. He arrived on the same day and gently examined my mother. She already started feeling better with only his presence. He then extracted from his medical bag a small needle and pricked her finger, letting a drop of blood fall on a glass side. In his customary laconic speech he said, "I will come back soon." Later that evening, Dr. Villalobos returned and told us, "*Doña* Celina has *paludismo* and here is some medicine for her," handing us a prescription for quinine. I was the designated errand boy and ran to the nearest drugstore, the *Botica Isabel*, and waited ten minutes for the pharmacist to fill out the prescription. After taking the quinine, my mother never experienced another attack of "migraine." Dr. Villalobos had cured her chronic, recurrent malaria, which she had probably acquired when, as a young woman, she had visited her brother's farm in Guanacaste, a northern province in Costa Rica, where mosquitoes and malaria were at the time rampant.

The admiration we already had for Dr. Villalobos was far surpassed after that experience. Many years later, I again encountered malaria in Panama and learned about the intricate life cycle of *Plasmodium falciparum*, which becomes dormant in the liver and then periodically showers the blood stream with countless schizonts, destroying red blood cells and causing shaking chills and fever, rendering its victims devoid of any energy to work and carry on their daily activities. Unlike yellow fever, falciparum malaria maims but does not kill the human host. In this sense, malaria has been more successful than yellow fever because it doesn't eliminate the human reservoir necessary for its existence and propagation.

The great American malariologist and pathologist, Samuel T. Darling, who worked in Panama during the construction of the canal (1904-1914), was one of the first to apply the *splenic index* to determine the incidence of malaria in large populations. Instead of obtaining blood smears and examining these microscopically for the presence of malaria parasites, a simple abdominal examination to detect splenomegaly (enlargement of the spleen) was practical and accurate enough to decide if mass treatment for malaria was necessary. It is possible that Dr. Villalobos' examination detected splenomegaly in my mother and this helped him to arrive at the correct diagnosis. Recurrent and chronic malaria not only causes splenomegaly but distinct calcifications as well which can be seen readily in a plain x-ray of the abdomen. The first time I saw this was in an abdominal x-ray my father-in-law brought for me to see in Panama.

The malaria parasite has the ability to develop resistance to antimalarial drugs. Drug-resistant malaria was first found in Southeast Asia during the Vietnam War and American soldiers brought it back to the United States. Chloroquine and amodiaquine no longer cured malaria and, as a result, quinine became the drug of choice at the time. Quinine, however, had several drawbacks. It is very bitter and William Gorgas reported that despite offering quinine free to all workers in the canal, many of the men spit out the tablets as they left the dispensary. A "turkey gobbler" loved to swallow the discarded tablets, only to develop later amblyopia (blindness) from quinine toxicity. Quinine also caused deafness. Despite these adverse side effects, the Isthmian Canal Commission freely dispensed forty thousand daily doses of quinine to canal employees at the peak of the canal construction. In order to make quinine more palatable and accessible, tonic water also was freely available. Tonic water had the equivalent of one tablet or five grains (325 mg) of quinine per ounce. This form of quinine remains today as the favorite accompaniment to gin, as in a "gin-and-tonic" cocktail. The only remaining question is: which type of gin do you prefer, Beefeater® or Tanqueray®?

Gorgas WC: *Sanitation in Panama*. New York: D. Appleton and Company, 1916.

20

CONCUSSION

Concussion is defined as a closed head injury associated with impaired level of consciousness and/or neurological function. Concussion is an important problem not only among professional athletes in boxing, hockey and soccer, but also in children playing team sports in school such as soccer and baseball. Lack of recognition of the possible consequences of concussion, especially in young children, may lead to more serious problems encompassed under the term post-concussion syndrome.

It is not necessary for the injury to require a direct blow to the head. A mother of an adolescent soccer player brought a cell-phone video recording showing the concussion her daughter had suffered and rendered her unable to function normally at home or at school. The camera captured clearly the impact of the two players as they jumped and collided trying to head the ball but the impact was on her chest, not her head. Neither is it necessary for the participant to lose consciousness in the aftermath of a concussion. The pathophysiology of concussion requires for the force of the impact to be translated to the brain, either directly or indirectly, in either an anteroposterior trajectory (whiplash) or as a rotational force with the neck turning in response to the pivotal force.

Since current neuroimaging tools such as CT or MRI are not sensitive enough to show any anatomical damage to the brain following a concussion, current explanations prefer to describe the consequences of concussion in terms of abnormalities in neurotransmitter function and abnormal influx of calcium into nerve cells. Although a chemical aberration may be part of the consequences of a concussion, the serious cumulative effect of repeated concussions and the prolonged disability (lasting as long as two years in some of our cases) suggest an anatomical lesion is more likely.

In shaken-baby syndrome, the mere shaking of the infant grabbed by the shoulders and resultant bobbing of the head back and forth due to the weak neck muscles, result in injury to the brain stem and this can be seen clearly in tissue preparations stained for axons (nerve endings) on microscopic examination. The shear forces disrupt the continuity of the axons and small hemorrhages are found in this vital part of the brain responsible for maintaining us alive.

I believe that a similar mechanism is at play in concussions. If mild, the subject recovers without any complications. However, if severe enough, the athlete may suffer neuropsychological complications manifested as poor concentration, memory, anxiety, and frequent headaches. The adolescent withdraws from social activities and becomes depressed. The headaches are worsened by mental and physical activity. Understandably, both the patient and parents are concerned and want reassurance that eventually their child will return to normal. It is important in these cases to obtain a detailed neuropsychological profile and follow advise to limit stress, both physical and mental activities. The children may require excessive amounts of sleep. They also require patience, understanding and support from all those around, reassuring them that everything is going to be all right at the end.

Preventive measures include the design of better protective helmets and baseline tests that can serve as points of reference for comparing brain function before and after concussion. Strengthening of the neck muscles with appropriate exercises may be wise, based on the higher incidence of concussion among female athletes who may have weaker neck muscles than males. Although headers in soccer, especially in younger children, are suspect and probably should not be permitted to be part of the game, the evidence available is not supportive. The maximum calculated speed of a soccer ball in flight is about thirty mph. In animal experiments, a speed of at least forty mph is necessary to cause a concussion.

The mechanisms responsible for post-concussion syndrome are not clear. Whatever these might be, it requires a very long time to repair itself. When headaches are frequent and disabling, administration of preventive therapy in the form of amitriptyline (a tricyclic antidepressant) may be helpful.

The current "epidemic" of concussions among school athletes has raised serious concerns and many questions. Hopefully, a better understanding of the mechanisms involved and the pathophysiology of post-concussion syndrome will spark serious research in both clinical and basic science, and provide better explanations to the many as yet unanswered questions about concussion.

21

PLAYING 'POSSUM

The call came from the Emergency Room as I was sitting in one of the examining rooms reviewing a patient's chart. "Your daughter was brought by ambulance because they were unable to wake her up. She is unresponsive. Please come at once!"

Most of us will carry moments like these as indelible in our memory for the rest of our lives: the death of a loved one, the first recorded videos of 9/11 or the shooting of a president in Dallas. Time seems to stop and events develop thereafter as if in slow motion, every frame captured in stunning detail, ready to be played over and over again as easily as clicking a remote control. Not only are the visual components captured and retained but also the emotional aspects that accompany the visual imagery, as if a sound track had been added to complete the cinematic experience.

I immediately left the office, my heart pounding loudly so that not only could I feel but hear the palpitations, rushing to find my car parked several blocks away. The distance from the clinic to the hospital was only a few miles long. The route had been traversed hundreds of times, so that figuratively one could drive with the eyes closed. But this time every corner, every street light, every traffic signal appeared to have slowed and tormented my haste to arrive at my destination, not knowing what I will find. As a neurologist, my thoughts are oppressive: Is my daughter in coma? Does she have meningitis or encephalitis? What if she has a ruptured brain aneurysm? But she is only eleven years old and this morning left for school as her usual ebullient, happy and hyperactive self.

At last I turn the corner and find the nearest parking spot to the Emergency Room. Now I run and enter the dreaded domain where many times before I have been called in the middle of the night to see a child who has had a neurological event, a convulsion, head trauma, poison ingestion, etc. I ask where Karen is and a nurse dutifully points to a cubicle obscured by a closed curtain. As I part the curtain, I see my daughter on a stretcher, breathing quietly, with no external signs of injury and peaceful. Unable to restrain myself and follow the engrained sequence expected from a neurology resident to obtain first a detailed history followed by a meticulous examination, I shout a single word that conveys my desperation, "Karen!" She immediately recognizes my voice and sits up like a bolt and answers me: "What?" At that moment my sense of relief obscures any reproach for causing me so much anguish, for the satisfaction of knowing that she is not seriously sick envelopes me with gratitude and my return to sanity. Then I ask, "What happened?" She answers simply, "I was sleepy and tired and didn't want anybody to bother me, so I went to sleep." The trip home was mostly a silent event. A continuation of mixed thoughts and emotions. The feeling of relief alternates but dominates the sense of reproach. We have always taught our children to be honest and sincere. How could this be? But then, Karen has not always followed conventional wisdom. We know she is different. Probably the most intelligent of our four children, but the one with the lowest scholastic performance. She is the one who evades her turn to do the dishes by suddenly leaving the dining table before we are finished with our meal, complaining of headache or abdominal pain, or promising her sister that she will pay her back if she will do her obligation today. I return to the clinic in a much better mood than when I left it a couple of hours before.

Since then, I have been called time and again to see a child who is unresponsive in the Emergency Department (the name has been changed from room to department just as other traditional names have been changed by those who have nothing better to do: medicine to health care; doctor to provider; patient to client; secretary to administrative assistant; etc.) After obtaining a detailed history and performing a thorough examination that fail to reach a convincing diagnosis, the possibility that the child (usually an adolescent), is feigning unresponsiveness begins to emerge as a more plausible explanation for the perplexing situation.

The unresponsive patient who is malingering will usually have both eyes closed but is attentive to all that is happening near by. It is not difficult to demonstrate to medical students and residents the "psychogenic" coma by simple techniques. "And now I will show you how this patient will wake up when I squeeze the 'cardiophrenic' nerve (no such thing) in the neck"; or, "Observe how the patient will open the eyes when I count to three." Less gullible adolescents will allow the examiner to lift an arm and let it fall by gravity to the side, but may not be smart enough to permit the limb to fall and hit the face and instead gently deviate it to the side. Pain is not usually useful in differentiating really impaired consciousness from hysterical coma, since patients will endure pinching, needlesticks, rubbing knuckles over the sternum and other pain-producing maneuvers probably invented during the Spanish inquisition and perpetuated by neurosurgeons to determine the level of consciousness. But the most useful technique I have learned over the years is to simply approach the patient and gently touch the eyelashes. The patient, not aware of what I am doing, will immediately blink, indicating he or she is awake, while the truly comatose patient will not respond. Repeating this maneuver will not work, as now the patient can anticipate the touching of the eyelashes and not respond by blinking. This easy and simple test has never failed to tell me if a patient is really unconscious or just attempting to mimic this state.

Among the most difficult dilemmas neurologists face is distinguishing true seizures from pseudoseizures. The highly touted measurement of prolactin levels to differentiate one from the other, although still used, appears to have no validity. The gold standard is not only expensive but time consuming: video-EEG monitoring. The latter requires for the patient to be admitted to an epilepsy monitoring unit, where electrodes are placed on the scalp to detect abnormal brain wave activity and a video camera records visually all the accompanying events. An adolescent who is having pseudoseizures will appear to have a convulsion with stiffening and then jerking of the body, but the EEG does not show the typical "spikes" (pointed or sharply-contoured brain waves) seen during most seizures. (One of the most experienced electroencephalographers used to explain a spike as "something that would hurt if you sit on it.")

Video-EEG documentation that the patient is having pseudoseizures is now sufficiently complicated to require a team of neurologists and psychiatrists to address the psychosocial factors that have evolved into pseudoseizures. Instead of making the patient and the parent feel guilty, pseudoseizures are now treated as any other neuropsychiatric disorder and given the attention it needs to rehabilitate the patient. Even in patients who have pseudoseizures, I have found the blink reflex to be helpful during the post-ictal (period of recovery after a seizure) period, as it may tell me that the patient is really fully awake and not totally or partially unconscious.

Charcot, the great French neurologist, was much interested in what he called "hystero-epilepsy" and during the Tuesday lessons at the Saltpêtrière in Paris (attended by not only doctors but intellectuals and socialites as well), Charcot, with the help of his pupils Josef Babinski and Gilles de la Tourette, would demonstrate women with pseudoseizures. It is said, although probably more of a myth or legend than a true event, that Charcot asked two of his famous students, Sigmund Freud and Josef Babinski, to find how to differentiate seizures from pseudoseizures. This motivated one to develop psychoanalysis and the other to discover the most famous sign in neurology, the plantar (Babinski) reflex. When unequivocally present, the Babinski response is indicative of a lesion in the pyramidal (corticospinal) tract and its absence proves the integrity of this important bundle of nerves that allows the brain to control one side of the body.

Today, sophisticated and expensive neuroimaging techniques have largely supplanted the clinical skills that allowed doctors at one time to diagnose difficult neurological problems. Neurologists continue to adhere to the traditional tools of observation, palpation and auscultation. To these must be added that of listening carefully to a detailed history. A good neurologist will arrive at the correct diagnosis most of the time before the results of additional tests are available. Some may regard these clinical skills in this day and age as anachronistic. We prefer to think of them as honoring the memory of those legendary clinicians who taught us how to use our brain and not allow it to become atrophied from disuse.

Neurologists are specialized in the study of the nervous system and its disorders. This represents perhaps the most complicated challenge to those who strive to alleviate suffering. Yet neurologists continue to address problems using the basic tools available to us: our hands, eyes, ears and brains.

22

STATUS EPILEPTICUS

To a neurologist, "status" means *status epilepticus*, a condition in which the patient has continuous seizures for a prolonged time or doesn't recover completely between seizures. This is a medical emergency because neurons in the brain become "exhausted" and die. Over the years, the time frame ascribed to status has decreased from twenty minutes in the 1950s to five minutes at present. Most seizures terminate spontaneously within five minutes so that, when they don't, it is more likely that the seizure will continue until terminated by pharmacological intervention or the cause of the seizures is removed.

The pharmacological treatment of status epilepticus has also evolved over time, but essentially consists of using two medications known as anticonvulsants or antiepileptic drugs (AED). These medications act by different mechanisms on the neuronal membrane excitability, making it less prone to become depolarized and discharge electricity (as a bolt of lightning, if you will). The amount of electricity discharged is measured in microvolts and in order to visualize the electrical discharges, these are magnified a million times so that they appear in the electroencephalogram (EEG) as spikes and waves. The spikes represent an abnormal, excessive electrical discharge by the cortical neurons, which is exactly the definition given by Sir Hughlings Jackson, a famous English neurologist, to a seizure more than one hundred years ago.

The two drugs of choice used to stop status epilepticus are phenytoin and phenobarbital. Both have been around for many years: phenytoin was introduced by Merritt and Putnam in 1938 and phenobarbital almost two decades earlier by Hauptmann in 1911. Phenytoin remains the most effective and widely used anticonvulsant in the world, although in children prolonged use causes undesirable cosmetic side effects that have limited its use. Phenobarbital usage has also decreased in children because of its effect on cognitive function. Nevertheless, when given intravenously, both are extremely effective in stopping status epilepticus. A more immediate anticonvulsant effect is obtained with the use of intravenous benzodiazepines. The latter agents are also very effective but may depress respirations. Over the years the favorite benzodiazepine has evolved also from diazepam to lorazepam, and now midazolam appears to be the favorite.

The call came to the hospital that Sarah, a young princess, was coming from the royal palace with seizures and to alert the child neurologist to be present in the Emergency Department for her arrival. As the doors of the hospital opened, a retinue of about twenty persons walked in briskly with anxious faces except for the young girl, who was obviously in status epilepticus and unresponsive. Heading the procession was an *imam* (religious leader) dressed in white and holding the Koran in one hand and a glass of water in the other, taking sips and spewing the water over the child, while pronouncing loud incantations from the sacred book.

I was taken aback by two factors. First, I didn't expect this demonstration of fervor by such a large group of believers and, second, I had learned by now to respect the cultural and religious idiosyncrasies of others. However, the crucial question in this scenario was how long to wait? Status epilepticus is a medical emergency and intervention should be implemented as soon as possible. How many minutes should I wait as a sign of respect? How many neurons are dying each minute while the religious ceremony continues? Finally, I step forward and start an intravenous route through which phenytoin is given and within minutes the princess ceases convulsing. Fortunately, a neurological examination shows no cognitive or motor deficits on the following day.

Sometimes we face situations when an important decision has to be made without delay. A good leader will usually decide immediately and worry later whether it was the right or wrong one. Decisions in medicine are more complicated and may carry dire consequences if not chosen correctly. Hence, some delay in reasoning or asking for help may be justified. The experience described still haunts me as I wrestled with the delay in intervening to stop status epilepticus in the young princess.

The dilemma between ancient beliefs and modern medicine still exists in many parts of the world. Mutual respect is an important requisite as alternative medicine has become part of the medical school curriculum. Many patients prefer herbal remedies and accupuncture to western medicine. We are careful now not to disparage homeopathy, chiropractic and other unconventional practices. I still believe that humility and respect are essential components in the practice of medicine. The most scientific and brilliant medical students do not make the best doctors. They often lack the humanism that bridges the gap between a healer and a sick person. There is no question in my mind that faith and confidence are imperative in the process of healing.

23

BRAIN DEATH

A member of the diplomatic corps was brought to the hospital accompanied by a parade of relatives, doctors and religious *imams*. The hospital authorities had been alerted and all department chairmen were anxiously waiting for the arrival of the official. At first glance it was obvious that he had been already dead for several hours. He had been brought to the hospital so that his official death would not appear to have taken place at the embassy.

The neurological examination disclosed that all brain function had ceased. The brain stem reflexes were absent and the patient was declared "brain dead." All good neurologists perform, in addition to a neurological examination, a general examination as well. To our surprise, the liver was markedly enlarged and firm consistent with cirrhosis. Earlier, a nasogastric tube had shown copious amounts of fresh blood in the stomach. It was then obvious that the patient had died of massive bleeding from esophageal varices (dilated veins) and cirrhosis (scarring) of the liver. This diagnosis was untenable in a place where religious restrictions prohibited the ingestion of alcohol. After hours of deliberation, the hospital administrators gathered all the chairmen and decided that the official diagnosis was a heart attack.

Neurologists are most familiar with the concept of brain death. For thousands of years, doctors have been called to declare that a patient has died. They search diligently for a pulse, listen to the heart, examine the pupils and then arrive at the undeniable conclusion that the individual is no longer alive. However, with the advent of mechanical ventilation and cardiorespiratory resuscitation, patients who otherwise would have died, now could be kept alive, if only artificially so. The definition of death required a revision. Since death had long been linked to departure of the soul from the body, the next step was to ask Pope Pius XII to formulate a modern definition of death that would encompass the new technical aspects of resuscitation. In an admirable example of wisdom, the spiritual leader declared that the definition of death was not a religious matter, but a medical matter and placed the ball right back on the doctors' court. Medical leaders accepted the challenge and formed a committee charged with the task of defining brain death. After much deliberation and hearing from many experts, an ad hoc committee from Harvard Medical School published in 1968 a landmark set of guidelines for defining brain death. Although these guidelines have been revised since, the intent remains essentially unchanged: a person is dead when brain function ceases.

A neurologist or competent doctor examines the brain stem reflexes and when none are found, the conclusion is irreversible brain death. The brain stem reflexes include the reaction of the pupils to light, the blink of the eyelids when the cornea is touched, the gag reflex when a tongue blade or catheter is pushed against the pharynx, the response of the eye movements to ice-water irrigation of the ear canals, the deep-tendon or muscle-stretch reflexes tested with a percussion hammer, response to deep-pain stimulus and respiratory effort when carbon dioxide accumulates. The presence of any one of these reflexes, whether absolute or equivocal, negates the state of brain death and the examination must be repeated twenty-four hours later. Although additional tests have been advocated to aid when the clinical evidence is not conclusive for brain death, such as brain wave (EEG) activity, cerebrovascular blood flow, arterial pulsations, etc., the clinical neurological examination remains the gold standard.

Unfortunately, a person who no longer has brain stem reflexes may still demonstrate what appear to be spontaneous, reflex or even volitional movements of the arms and legs. These confounding movements represent spinal reflexes which may be initiated by external stimuli and give the false appearance that the patient is still alive. This may require gentle but convincing explanations to otherwise incredulous relatives.

After the Harvard Ad Hoc Committee had established the parameters for brain death, an elderly practitioner wrote a letter to the *New England Journal of Medicine* complaining about the new guidelines. During his forty-year practical experience, he reported, he had pronounced dead hundreds of patients and none of them had ever come back alive! Now, here is a practical doctor with common sense I really admire.

A definition of irreversible coma. Report of the Ad Hoc Committee of the Harvard Medical School to examine the definition of brain death. *Journal of the American Medical Association* 1968; 205: 85-8.

24

RAGGEDY ANN

Despite my aversion to see or consult on medical problems among members of my own family, inevitably someone pleads for me to do exactly that. Over the years, I have come to believe that such requests are mainly motivated by a desire to determine my proficiency in medical matters, as my failures have easily exceeded any successes.

My mother, who was an encyclopedia of home remedies, often interrupted me when I, recently graduated from medical school, made some recommendation to the parents of a sick child in the neighborhood. Her pharmacopeia was centered on the liberal use of lemon juice for upper respiratory infections, dyspepsias, neuralgias and other ailments, some of which have apparently disappeared from our lexicon.

The word malaria (mal air) originated from the ancient belief that agues or fevers were caused by noxious vapors (miasmas) emanating from proximate swamps caused by decomposition of filth and vegetable matter. This belief is, however, still valid and ardently defended by members of my family, who keep admonishing me not to sit near a window or door because a cold draft may twist my neck or smite me with the fury of demonic spirits. Unfortunately, the scientific advances of Koch, Pasteur and Semmelweis have not undermined the entrenched wisdom of the miasmatic theory of disease in my family. To wit, my relatives still tie a handkerchief around the neck and insert cotton plugs impregnated with camphorated oil to ward off the poisonous drafts that surround them.

During one of our yearly trips to Panama and Costa Rica to visit our families, one of my wife's nephews brought his infant daughter, Marci, for evaluation of her developmental delay. Marci had been product of a normal pregnancy and delivery from a healthy mother, without any problems at birth. Her motor development, however, was at a standstill and they wanted to know why. A time and place was arranged for a neurological evaluation. Before Marci was placed on a sofa for examination, it was clear from simple observation what the problem was. She was as floppy as a rag doll and her head, trunk and extremities lay passively in her mother's arms as if she were a lifeless Raggedy Ann doll.

One of the first things we learn to do in pediatric neurology is the evaluation of a floppy infant, or as more accurately described in neurological terms, a hypotonic infant. The majority of these cases is due to an insult of the central nervous system during birth, most commonly hypoxia or birth asphyxia. In these cases, the hypotonia slowly evolves into spasticity and by two years of age the diagnosis becomes clear as cerebral palsy or spastic diplegia. Neurologists refer to these conditions as due to *upper* motor neuron (brain) injury. The rest (less than 20 percent) of the floppy infants have a *lower* motor neuron injury, that is, of the spinal cord, peripheral nerves, neuromuscular junction or muscle. These cases are more complicated, since additional studies are necessary to determine the etiology, including electrical tests of muscle function (EMG) or even a muscle biopsy.

In order to differentiate between upper and lower motor neuron injuries, neurologists then examine the muscle-stretch reflexes [deep-tendon reflexes (DTRs)] using a reflex hammer. Hammers come in different sizes and shapes. The three most commonly used are the "tomahawk" hammer which most medical students and residents use but only improperly; the Queen's Square (named for the National Hospital for the Paralyzed and Epileptic at Queen's Square in London) with its round head; and the Trömner hammer, which is a formidable weapon and weighs nearly a quarter pound despite its hollow handle and streamlined features. My Trömner hammer was presented to me as a gift when I completed my neurology residency, much as a disciple receives his sword when he has mastered the martial arts from his teacher. Although a Trömner reflex hammer is hard to misplace because of its considerable size, after several days of absence a mother called to tell me that she had inadvertently taken it home inside the diaper of her baby and, after thorough cleansing, would bring it back to my clinic—which she did.

But back to Marci, my floppy patient. When I tried to obtain her DTRs, none were to be found. This implied that it was not a brain injury but something else and that something else would require further complex and expensive testing, which I was reluctant to recommend. Trying to hide my discomfort, I rambled equivocally something akin to "hope and pray." What I said was that the motor delay was due to weak muscles and not to a brain injury and that it was better to wait and see how she developed with time. I could sense my discomfort as well as the disappointment of my relatives that not only did I not know what was wrong, but offered no treatment and much less a cure. What good were all those years dedicated to the study of the brain, when this highly touted specialist had no clear answers?

Marci slowly but surely started to make progress but it took a long time to achieve her motor milestones such as rolling over, sitting and walking. I was not asked again to repeat her neurological evaluation, such was the lack of confidence in my diagnostic abilities by her parents. The floppy infant is now in her 20s. She is a beautiful woman with plenty of suitors. I saw her dance salsa with her father and her feet were moving faster than my eyes could follow. If someone had told me twenty years before that the Raggedy Ann I saw then would look like this, I would not have believed it. Fortunately, Marci does not remember the time I saw her first and does not know about my feelings of despair then.

I have seen other babies like Marci since then. I still don't know the reason for the profound hypotonia. Perhaps it is due to delayed maturation of the white matter, but I have not been able to correlate this with appropriate brain MRI studies except in a few cases. Muscle biopsies are out of the question since most muscle diseases do not get better spontaneously. However, I have a cubbyhole to put these floppy babies and it is labeled "benign congenital hypotonia." The name is not that bad, as it sounds as if it is a real neurological disorder. The important part of the name is the "benign" part, which assures the parents that the condition is not serious and perhaps fully reversible. That is, unless the patient happens to be a relative of mine.

Gordon N: Benign congenital hypotonia: A syndrome or a disease. *Developmental Medicine and Child Neurology* 1966; 8: 330-335.

25

BROWN URINE

Brown urine may be caused by *myoglobinuria*, the presence in the urine of a muscle protein, myoglobin. Myoglobin may be released into the blood stream when muscle is injured or destroyed. If present in sufficient quantity, myoglobin will turn the color of the urine from yellow to red or brown. Myoglobinuria may be seen in chronic conditions such as muscle disorders when excessive exercise injures muscle. It can also occur in acute injuries such as motor vehicle accidents associated with crushing injuries affecting muscle. Large amounts of myoglobin may lead to renal failure, as the protein may obstruct the renal capillaries and interfere with normal kidney function.

The causes of myoglobinuria are varied and numerous. Apart from acute injuries, the most common cause is related to metabolic defects of muscle. Also known as inborn errors of metabolism (IEM), these defects include an important group of genetic defects involving mitochondria. Mitochondria are small cell organelles responsible for the production of energy in the cell. These tiny factories are thought to have been, at one time in the evolution of the cell, independent microorganisms much like bacteria, that eventually became incorporated in a symbiotic relationship with eukaryotic cells. Mitochondria consist of both DNA and RNA, but the genes encoding these are relatively few. Mitochondria have another peculiar and unique characteristic: they are transmitted to subsequent generations only by maternal lineage, that is, mitochondria are inherited only through the mother. Mitochondrial testing, therefore, can be used to determine genetic relationships between individuals and even ethnic groups. In the book *The Seven Daughters of Eve*, geneticist Bryan Sykes purported to show that by using mitochondrial analyses, maternal ancestry could be traced back all the way to Eve (of the Garden of Eden) and that her progeny formed seven distinct branches which represented our Western European ancestors.

Fifty years ago, only a handful of disorders were known to be due to mitochondrial defects. These were identified clinically by their presenting clinical features: subacute necrotizing encephalomyelopathy (SNE and also known as Leigh's disease, after Denis Leigh who described one of the earliest cases more than fifty years ago); progressive external ophthalmoplegia (PEO); ophthalmoplegia, retinitis pigmentosa and cardiomyopathy (Kearns-Sayre syndrome or KSS); Leber's optic atrophy (LOA); and mitochondrial myopathy, encephalopathy and lactic acidosis and stroke-like episodes (MELAS). Of these, the only one which affected younger children was Leigh's disease. The symptoms appeared early during the first or second year of life with abnormalities of respiration and developmental delay. As in many of the disorders of mitochondria, blood lactic acid and pyruvic acid levels were increased and it was thought that a certain ratio of these was more suggestive of Leigh's disease. The pathological findings in the brain were characteristic, showing injury (necrosis) in the basal ganglia, thalamus, brain stem and spinal cord, resembling but distinct from Wernicke's (alcoholic or thiamine deficiency) encephalopathy. With the advent of better neuroimaging techniques (CT and MRI), the characteristic changes in the brain were more easily recognized.

Because of the resemblance of the pathological findings in Leigh's disease to thiamine deficiency, the presence of a thiamine pyrophosphate (TPP) inhibitor was sought and found in tissues, blood and urine of Leigh's disease patients. This led to the development of a urine test by Jonathan Pincus at Yale University for a TPP inhibitor.

Twenty years later, neurologists interested in mitochondrial disorders, mainly at Columbia University in New York City, uncovered a whole new world of mitochondrial disorders, now requiring more sophisticated laboratory analyses on muscle biopsies or cultured skin fibroblasts. More than one hundred separate conditions are now listed in the On-line Mendelian Inheritance in Man (OMIM) database as mitochondrial disorders.

Returning to the subject of myoglobinuria, a patient who has muscle pain and weakness related to exercise or intercurrent illness may have one of several relatively rare diseases. These include carnitine palmitoyl transferase deficiency type II (CPT II); myophosphorylase deficiency (McArdle's disease or glycogen storage disease V); and phosphoglucomutase deficiency. A blood test called creatine phosphokinase (CPK or CK) will detect muscle injury (rhabdomyolysis) and urine analysis will disclose the presence of myoglobinuria. The presence of "ragged red fibers" in a muscle biopsy (so-called because the numerous abnormal mitochondria tend to stain red with trichrome stains and are distributed at the periphery of the muscle cell, giving it a ragged or "moth-eaten" appearance), also was helpful in detecting a mitochondrial disorder.

The past fifty years have witnessed the evolution of many genetic disorders as improved laboratory technologies have facilitated diagnosis. The clinical diagnosis has been improved, if not supplanted, by genetic testing. One important development has been that the old concept of one gene/one disease is no longer valid. We no longer accept that one phenotype (clinical presentation) is equivalent to one genotype (genetic defect). Many examples are now known to indicate that one genotype may give rise to several different phenotypes and, conversely, one phenotype may be the result of several different gene abnormalities. For example, Leigh's disease is now known to be caused by several different mitochondrial genes.

My interest in hereditary metabolic disorders (also known as inborn errors of metabolism) included mitochondrial disorders. Perhaps the most interesting mitochondrial disorder I have seen was brought to my clinic more than twenty years ago by a mother with two children, David and Donald, similarly affected with developmental delay, weakness and, later on, fatigue with exercise. After the limited investigations available at that time (including a muscle biopsy) were done, nothing diagnostic was found and the mother was advised that the children probably had a genetic disorder affecting mitochondrial metabolism but we had been unable to find the exact etiology.

Twenty-three years later, the mother brought David and Donald back to my clinic. I remembered her but not the children, as now they were adults after two decades had passed. This time she volunteered important new information. David, the older, had brown urine after exercise, although he was limited in the amount of exertion such as walking he could withstand before becoming completely exhausted. With this new information, I contacted a neuromuscular expert who had more experience with rare genetic myopathies. The differential diagnosis included those already mentioned above under myoglobinuria. An electrical test of muscle function (EMG) was not diagnostic. Both patients had been followed elsewhere since my departure from this area. Finally, blood samples were collected on both and sent for mitochondrial testing. To everyone's surprise, this showed a rare point mutation substituting adenosine for guanine in the mitochondrial RNA. A search in the literature revealed only a few reported cases of this mutation and the phenotype was not well characterized. At last, after more than two decades, a diagnostic enigma had been elucidated. As in many other cases, an established diagnosis did not help us to offer specific treatment or to prognosticate the future clinical course. Yet, the mother was grateful that, finally, she knew what was the matter with her children. And I was, too.

26

CANNIBALISM

Kuru is the name given by the aboriginal peoples of the Northern Highlands of New Guinea, the Fore, to a disease that was common among them, meaning unsteadiness. Because of their insularity and geographical isolation, little was known about the Fore until missionaries began to report about their first contacts with them.

The presence of what appeared to be an unknown neurodegenerative disease attracted the interest of Carleton Gajdusek, a neurologist from NIH, who befriended the Fore and spent time living among them. Gajdusek's initial epidemiological studies suggested that kuru was not hereditary and more likely was due to an environmental toxin. He obtained permission to autopsy kuru victims and managed to send tissue samples, especially from brain, to NIH for pathological, toxicological and viral studies. The latter included inoculation experiments in primates. For a number of years, nothing was found. Kuru became a mysterious disease.

Additional observations revealed that the Fore practiced endocannibalism. This practice followed their belief that the spirits of their ancestors could be preserved by ingestion of parts of their bodies. Women and children had priority over organs such as brain. The practice had been discouraged by authorities and missionaries, so that younger generations began to abandon it. Further epidemiological studies revealed that children and women were more affected than men and that the incidence of kuru was decreasing. At NIH, inoculated primates were kept under observation for years. Lo and behold, some of the experimental animals began to show signs resembling those of kuru many years later. Pathological examination of their brains showed similar findings to those found in kuru victims: a "swiss-cheese" destruction of brain tissue named *spongiform encephalopathy*. The novel concept began to emerge of a latent or slow virus with an incubation period of years, instead of days or weeks. The investigations on kuru yielded two Nobel prizes: one to Carleton Gajdusek for his work on kuru and later, to Stanley Prusinger for his demonstration that kuru and other spongiform encephalopathies (mad-cow disease and Jakob-Creutzfeldt disease) were caused by *prions*, new infectious agents different from bacteria, rickettsiae, viruses and other known infectious agents, that consisted only of replicating RNA segments. This revolutionized the concept of infectious diseases.

My introduction to this fascinating world of slow-virus diseases began when, as a neurology resident, I was the first to see and evaluate a prominent leader who had recently traveled to remote regions, including New Guinea. A few weeks after returning, he began to have difficulties with his cognitive functions, including speech. He then developed seizures characterized by subtle quick movements of his hands known as myoclonic seizures. An EEG showed abnormalities (PLEDS or periodic lateralized epileptiform discharges) that suggested the possibility of Jakob-Creutzfeldt disease, one of the spongiform encephalopathies, also known as J-C for short. After several months, death came mercifully to terminate such an agonizing and progressive neurological deterioration.

At autopsy, the pathological examination showed the "swiss-cheese" vacuolation of the brain characteristic of J-C disease and other transmissible spongiform encephalopathies. Those of us who were present at the autopsy were not aware that the disease could be transmitted through droplet and direct contact with mucous membranes, including eyes and mouth. Case reports documented the transmission of J-C disease by close contact, including by a corneal transplant in a prominent neurosurgeon. In our patient, the source of the infecting agent was unknown and his brief exposure to an endemic kuru region had nothing to do with his disease, since not enough time had elapsed to account for it.

Later on, human cases of mad-cow disease made all of us aware that rare disorders can become less rare and that geographical isolation no longer is a barrier to the dissemination of rare and unusual conditions in the world. The most amazing revelation to me is the realization that like us, all organisms—even the most minute—adapt to the environment in order to survive. In most situations, we are only innocent bystanders and not the primary hosts for these parasites, if I may be permitted to use this word to designate all those living organisms that may live inside our bodies. I believe that parasites will always accompany us in our journey to the future. They represent our companions, whether we like it or not.

Liberski PP: Historical overview of prion disease: A view from afar. *Folia Neuropathologia* 2012; 50: 1-12.

Grabow JD, Campbell RJ, Okazaki H, et al: A transmissible subacute spongiform encephalopathy in a visitor to the eastern highlands of New Guinea. *Brain* 1976; 99: 637-58.

27

HAND MOVEMENTS

Until Andreas Rett, a developmental pediatrician in Austria, recognized a syndrome characterized by autism, microcephaly and purposeless hand movements in the early 1950s, no one seemed to be aware of this entity.

The anecdotal account I heard was that Rett was the only pediatrician in Vienna who saw all the handicapped children in his clinic. The patients were lined up in a long corridor flanked by two benches. One day, as he walked by the corridor leading to his office, he noted a young girl who was making some unusual movements with her hands. The latter resembled hand-washing movements. As he walked down the corridor some more, he saw another girl with the same purposeless repetitive hand movements. He stopped and asked the mother if her daughter and the other girl on the far side of the bench were related. She said "no." He then made a mental note and before he was done, he had collected a number of these patients. His first publication was in the voluminous *Handbook of Neurology*, published by Elsevier and which consisted of more than one hundred volumes encompassing all that was known in neurology at the time. Rett had done some studies and had found increased blood ammonia in his patients. But it was not until he teamed up with his Swedish and French counterparts and together published a seminal paper in the *Annals of Neurology* in 1983, describing thirty-five patients with similar clinical characteristics, that the disorder became better recognized. Following this publication, most of us realized that we had seen one or more similar patients in our clinic. Rett syndrome became universally known.

One of the youngest patients with Rett syndrome I met was Margaret, a three-year-old girl whose behavior I could not explain. Every three months Margaret was brought by her mother to see me and each time she cried inconsolably, from the moment she saw me until she left the examining room. I had never before had that negative experience with any of my patients. After one or two visits, at the most, those young children were able to recognize me and the surroundings. I had always prided myself of being able to put young children and infants at ease and usually completing an examination was an easy task. But not with this child. The mother and I wondered why Margaret didn't warm up to me, until a year or more later, when she began to show the unmistakable purposeless, repetitive hand movements, autistic behavior and head growth deceleration. Her antagonistic behavior was due to Rett syndrome. Uncontrollable crying is one of the early signs of Rett syndrome.

Rett syndrome became one of the most common causes for developmental delay in young girls, perhaps due to its easy clinical recognition. During my six years in the Middle East, Rett syndrome was so frequently seen in the clinic that the nurses would tell me the diagnosis before I had a chance to examine the patients. This high incidence was related to the prevalent high consanguinity: at least 80 percent of all parents in the clinic were first or second cousins.

One of the most brilliant pediatric neurologists, Hoda Zoghbi, was able to explain the cause of Rett syndrome. Trained under Marvin Fishman in Dallas, Zoghbi studied the molecular genetics of Rett syndrome in her research laboratory at Baylor. As often happens, serendipity played an important role in the discovery that Rett syndrome was caused by defect in one of the methylation genes, *MeCP2*. When Zoghbi presented her findings at one of the annual neurology meetings, we were dazzled by the impeccable methods and results, including a "knock-out" mouse model of Rett syndrome, in which ablation of the responsible gene resulted in similar autistic features, with typical "hand washing" movements *in mice*!

But why does Rett syndrome affect only females? In several other disorders, usually called X-linked, the gene defect resides in the X-chromosome. Since females have only one X-chromosome, while males have one X and one Y sex chromosome, the female is the affected one. Males may not survive the "double" abnormality and die in utero or shortly after birth. Due to a phenomenon labeled as the Lyon hypothesis, one of the sex chromosomes may be "deactivated" and a male may be born with true Rett syndrome. Such cases are few and far in between but well documented in the literature, as in male Turner syndrome. Not all Rett syndrome patients have the genetic defect described by Zoghbi. Several other genetic defects have been found and in some the clinical features vary somewhat from the typical Rett syndrome. Hence the name given to these as examples of "atypical Rett syndrome."

Thanks to the observational abilities of Andreas Rett and the groundbreaking research of Huda Zoghbi, Rett syndrome is now diagnosed early and appropriate supportive treatment made available to these patients.

Hagberg B, Aicardi J, Dias K, et al: A progressive syndrome of autism, dementia, ataxia, and loss of purposeful hand use in girls: Rett's syndrome: a report of 35 cases. *Annals of Neurology* 1983; 14: 471-9.

Shahbazian MD, Zoghbi HY: Rett syndrome and MeCP2: Linking epigenetics and neuronal function. *American Journal of Human Genetics* 2002; 71: 1259-72.

28

HEATSTROKE

The history of heatstroke goes back centuries to the time when military campaigns were waged in unfamiliar territories. British soldiers, for example, marched under the searing sun, wearing the helmets and thick uniforms that kept them from dissipating body heat, resulting in excess casualties from heatstroke.

Curiously, heatstroke seldom happens in acclimated populations who have learned to protect themselves from the heat by covering under many layers of clothing. Although epidemics of heatstroke have been reported in the past during the pilgrimage to Mecca, preventive measures such as abundant drinking water and air conditioning have kept the number of casualties down.

More recently, a heat wave in France resulted in thousands of deaths, mostly among the elderly and sick, who lacked air conditioning or transportation to cooler environments. In Chicago, a heat wave in 1991 also brought a high mortality to the inhabitants housed in apartment complexes without proper ventilation.

Heatstroke is defined as a condition in which the core temperature rises above 104 degrees Fahrenheit (40° C) and the person has neurological signs such as disorientation progressing to delirium and coma. The mortality is high and treatment consists of heroic measures to lower the core temperature by infusing cold intravenous solutions, enemas and cooling of the skin by conduction and/or evaporation. Lack of rapid implementation of cooling measures leads to a catastrophic cascade of physiological events, marked by the release of acute inflammatory cytokines, which can cause further tissue damage. The most important injury site involves the lining (endothelium) of the intestines and other organs.

Hyperthermia differs from heatstroke by the absence of neurological symptoms. In that sense, fever is a common example familiar to all of us. Fever is produced when an invading agent injures tissue and releases the same cytokines that are operative in heatstroke, but without the catastrophic consequences. One of my pediatric professors thought fever should not be treated, since it is a protective physiological mechanism against infection. Fever, however, may cause seizures in one out of every twenty children before the age of four to six years and, therefore, justifies treatment with antipyretic agents such as aspirin, acetaminophen or ibuprofen. I must confess that at one time we used ice water admixed with alcohol to bathe infants and young children with high fevers. This practice is no longer acceptable. We learned then that chills announced the "breaking" of the fever or what is referred to in medical terms as *lysis*.

The beneficial effects of fever at one time led to the treatment of syphilis with malaria. The organism responsible for syphilis, *Treponema pallidum*, is sensitive to high body temperatures and this type of treatment gained popularity at the turn of the Twentieth Century before arsenic compounds and later penicillin became more effective forms of treatment.

Experimental studies by a colleague, Abderrezak Bouchama, using a colony of baboons have helped to elucidate the pathophysiology of heatstroke. Genetic predisposition results in a critical complication, malignant hyperthermia, when certain susceptible patients are given halothane or other related volatile anesthetics. The potentially fatal precipitous rise in body temperature and muscle contractions may be counteracted with the prompt administration of dantrolene. Rhabdomyolisis, myoglobinuria and marked elevations of the muscle enzyme creatine phosphokinase (CPK) in the blood are consequences of malignant hyperthermia. A hereditary predisposition to malignant hyperthermia may be identified with genetic testing for the *ryanodine* gene *RYR1*, especially if there is a family history of intolerance to volatile anesthetics and succinylcholine.

When I developed pneumonia as a child, hot plasters of "antiphlogistines" were applied to my chest. Although I survived, keloid scars remain to remind me that even today, mustard and similar plasters are still used to treat inflammation and other ailments. Phlogiston was the putative component of air that was responsible for burning of flammable materials until oxygen was discovered by Priestley in 1774. This discovery marked the end of alchemy and the beginning of modern chemistry. Despite many advances in modern medicine, plasters, poultices and purgatives remain popular among those who still believe in the four humours of Aristotle and Galen.

Bouchama A, Knochel JP: Medical Progress: Heat Stroke. *New England Journal of Medicine* 2002; 346: 1978-88.

Bouchama A, Dehbi M, Chaves-Carballo E: Cooling and hemodynamic management in heatstroke: Practical recommendations. *Critical Care* 2007; 11: R54.

29

WEAR-AND-TEAR PIGMENTS

The patient presented to the attending physician was Jonathan, a twelve-year-old lad who had developed progressive loss of vision, a decline in cognitive abilities and seizures. The attending accompanied me to see the patient and after examining him, took me back to his office and said, "The patient has Batten's disease." I had no idea what he meant and patiently he told me who Batten was and then about the disease that bears his name, now called by the tongue-twister *neuronal ceroid-lipofuscinosis* or NCL.

Fred Batten (1865-1918) was a neurologist at Queen's Square Hospital for the Paralyzed and Epileptic in London. He had a special interest in childhood neurological disorders, particularly cerebellar diseases. In one of his experimental studies on ataxia, he removed the cerebellum from cats and then dropped them for a distance to see if they could still land on their feet. Although the subspecialty of child neurology did not exist as such at the time, Batten wrote one of the first chapters on neurological diseases in children and, therefore, vies with Bernard Sachs as the anointed "father of pediatric neurology."

Among Batten's publications is his report on a progressive degenerative disorder of the nervous system characterized pathologically by the accumulation of pigments in the brain called ceroid and lipofuscin. Both of these pigments result from injury or death of tissue and have the physical property of autofluorescence under ultraviolet light, making their identification in pathological tissues relatively easy. Extensive pathological studies had identified three different variations of the disorder, separated mainly according to age at onset. Each was given an eponymic designation based on those who described them initially: Santavuori-Haltia for the infantile type; Spielmeyer-Vogt for the juvenile type; and Kuf disease for the adult type. Some preferred to designate as Batten's disease the juvenile form.

In 1969, Paul Dyken, who had studied one of the largest series of these patients, coined the term neuronal ceroid-lipofuscinosis or NCL, to satisfy those who disliked eponyms and preferred a descriptive name for neurological disorders. With time, NCL displaced the confusing terminology that had existed before.

After reading and learning about Batten's disease, I reviewed all the cases that had been seen previously at our hospital and presented this information at grand rounds Although I had also written a full-length article about these cases, this was not published.

Other than based on the clinical features of the patients, NCL could be diagnosed by demonstrating the presence of the ceroid-lipofuscinosis pigments using electron microscopy of brain biopsies. These pigments had varied peculiar morphological features that resembled fingerprint, curvilinear and granular bodies. Fortunately, these inclusion bodies were also found in more accessible tissues such as skin, mucous membranes and white blood cells. The latter afforded an easy but treacherous method for diagnosis, as it required a pathologist versed in interpretation of electron microscopic examinations of biopsies. Lack of an experienced pathologist willing to patiently examine the ultrastructural morphology of white blood cells in suspected patients could result, unfortunately, in false negative reports.

In the upper Midwest of the United States there is an increased incidence of NCL. This can be traced to Scandinavian ancestries and epidemiological studies in the Västerbotten region of Sweden suggest the presence of a "founder" effect, that is, an individual from whom most cases are derived and inherited in an autosomal recessive manner. This means that each parent has one of the corresponding genes and in that case, one out of four offspring may be so affected, while the parents and children with only one "bad" gene do not manifest the disease.

Batten's disease is also very common in the Middle East due to consanguinity (frequent marriage between first and second cousins), so that with the help of electron microscopy and a sample of peripheral blood, the diagnosis could be confirmed most of the time. Unfortunately, there was and still there is no cure for NCL and treatment is mainly supportive, including control of the seizures, which was accomplished in most cases with the use of vigabatrin.

With the advent of molecular genetics, studies by Kristina Wisniewski at the New York Institute for Basic Research in Brain Disabilities, identified the responsible genes and the classification evolved from phenotype (based on clinical features such as age and symptoms) to genotype. Our knowledge of Batten's disease has greatly expanded since Batten's initial description of the ailment. I favor using his name, as I find it easier to pronounce correctly than the more awkward neuronal ceroid-lipofuscinosis. Batten also reminds us that the pioneers who first became interested in neurological disorders of children should not be forgotten.

Chaves-Carballo E: Eponym: Frederick E. Batten: Father of pediatric neurology. *Southern Medical Journal* 1978; 71: 1428-9.

Dyken, PR: The neuronal ceroid lipofuscinosis. *Journal of Child Neurology* 1989; 4: 165-74.

Wisniewski KE, Kida E, Golabek AA, et al: Neuronal ceroid lipofuscinosis: Classification and diagnosis. *Advances in Genetics* 2001; 45: 1-34.

30

RED LOBSTER

Audrey, an intelligent fifteen-year-old young lady, began to have episodes characterized by feeling dizzy, headaches and turning "red as a lobster". I had not previously encountered such a colorful description of a patient's symptoms.

I recalled as a medical student when a general practitioner in Oklahoma administered monthly injections of vitamins to his patients, who became flushed and turned red, feeling much better after each treatment. I also recalled the "hot flashes" experienced by women during menopause. Could Audrey have some hormonal imbalance that would trigger the unusual paroxysmal events she described? Other rare disorders came to mind such as carcinoid syndrome, in which a tumor secretes a substance that causes vasodilatation and tachycardia. I remembered analyzing urine in the laboratory for 5-hydroxyindoleacetic acid, or 5-HIAA, looking for evidence of this disorder. Another possibility was porphyria, of which there are several different types with different clinical manifestation, but one of which (porphyria cutanea tarda) may be skin sensitivity to sunlight manifested as rashes and blisters. These rare disorders would be discussed from time to time in the differential diagnosis of clinicopathological cases presented in the *New England Journal of Medicine*. But rare cases are found only rarely (as one may wisely surmise) and in the day-to-day operations the old adage remains valid: "when one hears hoofbeats, don't think of zebras, think of horses." However, I could not think of any horses when trying to explain the etiology of this patient's skin color turning red as a lobster.

One of the useful lessons when dealing with strange or unusual cases is to verify that the patient is accurate in describing the symptoms. Neurologists are quite proficient in this skill and will spend considerable time dissecting in detail each component of the complaint. Is the color of the skin red or purple? Does the color change start in the head and then spread to the rest of the body? Do you feel hot or cold? Is there an associated diaphoresis (excessive sweating)? Does your heart beat fast (palpitations)?

The decision was made to admit Audrey and observe for any recurrence of these episodes. Within a few hours came the report from the ward that Audrey was having one of the paroxysmal events and, sure enough, she was red as a lobster! All vital signs remained normal and routine laboratory tests were also unremarkable. The possibility was entertained that this could be some unusual type of epileptic seizure and an electroencephalogram (EEG) study was obtained. This showed epileptiform discharges from the occipital region. A video-EEG was then requested to try to record the brain waves during one of these episodes and document that these were truly seizures. However, as frequently happens, Audrey did not have any more events during these recordings.

When we talk about the nervous system, neurologists refer mainly to two components: the central nervous system (brain, cerebellum, brain stem and spinal cord) and the peripheral nervous system (nerves). There is a third component, sometimes overlooked, and that is the *autonomic nervous system*. The diseases of the autonomic nervous system affecting children that we saw as medical students and residents were few and far in between. There was Riley-Day syndrome, a genetic disorder more common among Eastern European Ashkenazi groups, manifested by skin discoloration, smooth tongue due to a relative absence of fungiform papillae and diminished sweating, lacrimal secretions and saliva. Occasionally, we would do a sweat test using iodine and starch to map out on the skin areas with decreased sweat production or inject subcutaneously histamine and observe the resultant triple response: redness, flare and wheal, that indicated an intact histaminic reaction. Another diagnostic test was instilling methacoline drops in the eye and observing the pupillary response. I must confess that despite looking for Riley-Day cases periodically, I was unable to confirm the diagnosis in a single instance.

More recently, however, a new autonomic disorder has emerged and our initial experience suggests that this may be more common than anticipated. Patients usually complain of headache, dizziness and vague symptoms, which may suggest anxiety or stress-related phenomena. This new disorder is named *postural orthostatic tachycardia syndrome*, or POTS.

Orthostatic hypotension is the inability of the autonomic nervous system to compensate rapidly to changes in posture. This is commonly seen in elderly populations as well as in young, tall and slender individuals who experience light-headedness when getting up too quickly from a sitting position. Measuring blood pressure and pulse while supine (laying flat), sitting and standing will show more than thirty pulse beats difference, indicating poor autonomic response in POTS. The use of midodrine, an alpha-agonist, or of fludrocortisone, a fluorinated corticosteroid, may promptly and effectively suppresses the symptoms in many of these patients.

Autonomic disorders remained a curiosity and "zebras" in our collective medical encyclopedia until Phil Low at the Mayo Clinic began his lifelong studies of the autonomic nervous system. As in many other obscure areas of medical practice, Low began by developing basic tests to measure the function of this neglected system. His text *Disorders of the Autonomic Nervous System* became the foremost authority on the subject. As an aside, it is of interest that three clinicians from the same department in a small mid-western town became the world's experts in three important fields of neurological endeavor: Peter Dyck in peripheral neuropathies; Andy Engle in myopathies; and Phil Low in autonomic disorders. To be selected as a neurology resident and to learn from these three giants was, indeed, a privilege.

The definition of an epileptic seizure was given to us over a hundred years ago by Hughlings Jackson, who worked with William Gowers at the venerable Hospital for the Paralyzed and Epileptic at Queen's Square in Great Ormond Street, London. According to Jackson, a seizure is the sudden electrical discharge of a group of neurons from the cerebral cortex. This definition seemed to exclude the possibility that seizures could originate in the autonomic nervous system, as part of it is distributed outside the brain in autonomic ganglia and nerve bundles near the spinal cord. However, autonomic symptoms may accompany epileptic seizures. These symptoms include flushing, tachycardia, diaphoresis (excessive sweating) and vomiting.

Henri Gastaut, a French epileptologist, was among the first to describe seizures manifested mainly by autonomic features and correlated these with occipital or posterior epileptiform discharges. More recently, a Greek epileptologist, C.P. Panayiatoupoulos, described not only one but several more types of autonomic seizures and these have become known as Panayiatoupoulos syndrome. The fact that these types of seizures are rare makes the diagnostician uneasy about the accuracy of the diagnosis. The next step is to review the literature on the subject, followed by consultations with experienced epileptologists. This was done with experts from Boston Children's Hospital, who agreed with Audrey's diagnosis.

In the absence of a diagnostic test, a practical approach is to treat the patient with anticonvulsants to see if the paroxysmal attacks respond favorably or not. Once this was done, Audrey stopped having the red lobster episodes and was able to return to school and resume her normal activities.

Panayiotopoulos CP: *A Clinical Guide to Epileptic Syndromes and their Treatment.* London: Springer, 2010.

31

VERTIGO

My wife, a retired nurse, loves to be near patients and hospitals. After she was unable to do bedside nursing because of two vertebral fractures caused by osteoporosis, she continued to work part-time as an interpreter and then as a patient representative. While walking the long corridors in the hospital, she noted that certain neck maneuvers made her dizzy and she avoided looking up or to her extreme sides. The dizziness was not light-headedness but vertigo, the type where things start moving around you and accompanied by a feeling of instability and at times nausea. She adapted to this condition, which was more of a nuisance than a disability.

On one lucky day, as she was coming out of the hospital elevator, the sudden stop of the contraption invented by Otis, caused her to experience a sudden onset of vertigo and she braced herself against the wall to keep from falling. Behind her a gentle voice asked, "Can I help you? Are you dizzy?" My wife answered apologetically that she suffered from these paroxysmal episodes of vertigo. The helping voice came from a physical therapist who had been working for many years at the same hospital. She waited a few minutes until my wife felt better and said, "Come with me to P.T." She then explained that these episodes of vertigo were due to a problem in her vestibular apparatus, where the small concretions (tiny grains of sand) called otoconia were displaced from their usual location and fell into another place in the semicircular canals, producing vertigo. She had seen many similar patients in the past and had performed a simple canalith repositioning maneuver which usually helped or completely eliminated the paroxysmal attacks of vertigo.

The repositioning maneuver, sometimes called the Hallpike-Turner maneuver, consists of placing the person on an examination table and while sitting up, suddenly moving the trunk and head backwards so that the head rests at a lower level than the body and the neck is turned to one side. This will reproduce the same feeling of vertigo and abnormal jerking eye movements (nystagmus) toward the side of the inner ear that is characteristic of benign paroxysmal or positional vertigo. The Hallpike-Turner maneuver is an attempt to relocate the tiny grains into a sac-like structure called the utricle where they no longer are capable of producing vertigo. Most patients recover after one or two maneuvers. If the vertigo later returns, this exercise can be repeated as often as necessary. My wife had no more vertigo for several months until she began to experience a couple of slight ones and a return visit to her physical therapist solved the problem.

Benign paroxysmal vertigo (BPV) in children and benign paroxysmal positional vertigo (BPPV) in adults are quite common, disabling and frightening. Yet the treatment is simple and effective. I had learned about it as a neurology resident but failed to diagnose and treat it correctly in a member of my own family. Doctors who attempt to evaluate and treat close relatives or friends are at risk of falling into this same trap. The emotional and/or genetic attachment to the patient clouds one's judgment and results in loss of objectivity. This may lead to errors of omission or commission that may be costly. For this reason, I believe a doctor should avoid ministering to his or her own family.

Olivia, one of my granddaughters, is one of the brightest persons I know. She loves to read books and has quite an analytical mind. At age twelve, she constantly surprises us with her maturity, musical abilities and her endless sympathy for handicapped persons. I think she is destined to study medicine, although she doesn't know this yet.

Olivia began to have episodes of benign paroxysmal vertigo (BPV) before she was one year old. These were no ordinary episodes of vertigo. She would get sick enough to have repeated emesis and had to lie still for hours until the vertigo subsided. Sometime in the course of these events, she began to complain also of headaches and she was diagnosed by her pediatrician as having "abdominal migraine." I thought that what she had was benign paroxysmal vertigo as a childhood migraine equivalent. Referral to one of the senior and most respected pediatric neurologists in the country confirmed the clinical diagnosis. I had the opportunity to witness by myself an associated phenomenon only rarely reported in children with BPV: abnormal and chaotic eye movements (opsoclonus).

Children with neurological problems can be interesting and baffling at the same time. Migraine is common in children, but when it manifests at an early age, there may not be any accompanying headache. The absence of a headache can confound even experienced pediatricians and the diagnosis of childhood migraine missed altogether. It is only after a detailed history reveals the strongly positive family history of migraine, usually affecting females on the mother's side, and the appearance of more typical migraine attacks several years later, that the correct diagnosis is then confidently made.

There are at least five well-known "migraine equivalents" in children. The first and more common I already have described above: BPV. A second migraine equivalent is sometimes also called abdominal migraine but I dislike the term and have disparaged its use by explaining to medical students and residents that, as far as I know, there is no brain tissue in the abdomen. The second type of childhood migraine presents with repeated bouts of vomiting but differs from cyclic vomiting in the predictable periodicity and protracted vomiting seen in the latter. Cyclic vomiting often leads to visits to the Emergency Department for treatment of dehydration with intravenous fluids, as well as administration of antiemetics to stop the vomiting and a hypnotic to induce restful sleep.

A third type of migraine equivalent in children, and perhaps the least common, is the so-called Alice-in-Wonderland syndrome. This is characterized by metamorphopsia, that is, mainly visual hallucinations in which a part of the body gets bigger or smaller. The last patient with this ailment I saw in the clinic only a couple of months ago. An intelligent five-year old, explained to me: "My arm starts to get longer and longer and things it is trying to reach get smaller and smaller." Lewis Carroll (a pseudonym for Charles Dodgson), the author of *Alice in Wonderland*, was a migraneur and it is believed that some of his ideas for the book came from his own experiences with migraine attacks.

Most migraine patients have a type A personality and perform well in school (if not straight As) and are involved in multiple extra-curricular activities, including sports (soccer, swimming), music (piano lessons, band, choir), arts (dancing, ceramics, painting) and community services (church, scouts, raising funds for worthy causes). Migraine victims handle a dangerous schedule full of activities. I was not surprised to find that Olivia, my granddaughter, had a computer-generated list of her daily schedule starting with waking up early, taking a shower, brushing her teeth, dressing, eating breakfast, etc. Each one of these daily activities was allotted a certain number of minutes. Such a stressful schedule may be detrimental, since although migraine has a strong genetic component, stress contributes to make migraine attacks more frequent and severe. My advise to migraine patients and their parents is to make a list of activities in order of importance and begin to eliminate those at the bottom of the list until the headaches improve. Often the child is relieved just to know that his or her parental expectations are not as demanding as they once were.

A fourth type of migraine equivalent is vertebro-basilar migraine. This appears to be more common in adolescent girls who complain of dizziness, poor balance that makes walking difficult, and perhaps other brain stem signs that help to localize the site of neurological dysfunction.

A fifth and last type of childhood migraine is probably more common in adults. This is known as acute confusional migraine. The victim becomes confused, disoriented and distraught by finding him or herself in a strange place among unrecognizable people. Although this might seem difficult to differentiate from certain epileptic seizures such as complex partial seizures in which feelings of *déjà vu* or *jamais vu* represent an altered level of consciousness, seizures rarely last longer than three to five minutes, while migraines usually have a duration of several hours.

The advent of functional magnetic resonance studies (fMRI) has helped us to understand better the pathophysiology of migraine. The aura that presages an attack of migraine may be in the form of visual phenomena such as spots (scotomas) which are moving or stationary, bright (scintillating) or dark, zigzag (pallisading, fortification spectra) forms, or involve small or large portions of the visual fields. Auras have long been explained by constriction or narrowing of the vascular supply to specific regions of the brain concerned with vision (occipital lobes). The headache that typically follows the aura was also explained as due to vasodilatation (enlargement of the blood vessels) in which the small nerves in the arterial walls (vasa nervorum) are stretched and this generates pain signals to the brain. The vascular pathophysiology of migraine was supported by the beneficial response to treatment with ergot derivatives (vasoconstrictors) early at the onset of the migraine attack.

However, functional MRI studies of individuals during an attack of migraine revealed a phenomenon that had been described as a curiosity many years ago by a Brazilian neurophysiologist. While recording the electrical activity of the brain in rabbits, Aristides de Leão observed a slowly moving or spreading wave of depressed electrical discharges from the surface of the brain. This became known as the "cortical depression of Leão" and remained a curiosity until it was found more recently in several patients during an attack of migraine. This phenomenon raises more questions than answers about the pathophysiology of migraine. How does the cortical depression of Leão relate to the initial aura and the pain that follows in migraine? Is this phenomenon also present in children with migraine or migraine equivalents?

A holistic approach to the treatment of migraine in children requires a dedicated team of experts. Pain management not only requires analgesics (never opiates or narcotics) but also behavioral psychology to teach the patient to cope with pain and not become its victim. Preventive medication (beta-blockers and tricyclic antidepressants) has been shown to be at least 80 percent effective in controlled studies and is the cornerstone of pharmacological approach. The use of newer medications such as triptans is more useful to terminate a migraine attack when it has already started. However, these are not as well tolerated in children and even in adolescent patients adverse side effects may be a limiting factor. Herbal and other alternative compounds are commonly used when traditional medications are ineffective. Their easy accessibility without need for a prescription and the well-known placebo effect in migraine (about 40 percent) must be balanced with the fact that quality control of these medication is not supervised by FDA and that the only legal requirement by the government is that these should cause no harm. In a few cases, controlled studies have shown efficacy of several unconventional or alternative treatments. Newer evidence-based guidelines for the treatment of migraine have added several herbals, vitamins and minerals to the arsenal of effective preventive agents: butter-burr, feverfew, riboflavin and magnesium. Caffeine has a long tradition in the treatment of migraine. Time-honored preparations included APC (aspirin/acetaminophen, phenacetin and caffeine) and Fiorinal® (butabalbital, aspirin and caffeine), and others. A colleague frequently prescribed a cup of coffee for children with migraine, convinced of its efficacy. In coffee-producing countries such as Brazil, Colombia and Costa Rica, coffee consumption starts early, sometimes before the age of five years. It would be interesting to know if epidemiological studies show that the incidence of migraine is less in these countries than in the United States. This would have to be followed by additional studies to demonstrate if Folgers® is better for migraine than Maxwell House® or Starbucks®.

American Academy of Neurology: Evidence-based guideline update: NSAIDs and other complementary treatments for episodic migraine prevention in adults. *Neurology* 2012; 78: 1346-53.

American Academy of Neurology: Evidence-based guideline update: Pharmacologic treatment for episodic migraine prevention in adults. *Neurology* 2012; 78: 1337-45.

32

MUSCLE WEAKNESS

Guillaume Benjamin Amand Duchenne de Boulogne (1806-1875) is considered to be the father of French neurology, as he inspired Jean-Martin Charcot, the greatest neurologist in France, to become interested in this nascent field. Whereas Duchenne was "unworldly, naïve, absent-minded and inarticulate," Charcot emerged and surpassed his mentor with his observational and organizational skills.

Duchenne was indefatigable and scoured the wards of all the larger Paris hospitals searching for neurological cases. His interest in the application of faradic (direct) electrical currents to stimulate muscles led him to pioneer contributions in the study of neuromuscular diseases. Among these, of course, was his discovery of the progressive muscular dystrophy that bears his name. Charcot, who had first described multiple sclerosis, asked himself (as many others), "How is it that, one fine morning, Duchenne discovered a disease which probably existed in the time of Hippocrates?"

In 1862, Duchenne described in a short paper the pseudohypertrophic type of muscular dystrophy. Later he studied the degenerative changes in muscle biopsies obtained from these patients. His contemporary, Gowers, added the classic sign or maneuver, in which an affected child attempts to arise from the floor by using his legs as climbing poles, as if walking on himself. Thanks to funding raised every year by the Jerry Lewis Telethon, research in neuromuscular diseases has facilitated the diagnosis and treatment of muscular dystrophy.

DMD is inherited as an X-linked disorder. The mother carries the abnormal gene that produces the protein *dystrophin* and, even though she herself remains unaffected, half of her children will inherit DMD. When I went to the Middle East, I was not surprised to see my first case of DMD in Hamed, a boy with enlarged calves, waddling gait and a positive Gowers' sign. After trying to explain that the weakness was not the result of any indiscretion or abuse by the child, but an inherited problem, the father asked directly, "Who is responsible for transmitting the disease: the mother or the father?" Before I realized where he was heading, I answered that the mother carried the defective gene. At a follow-up visit six months later, the father returned alone with the boy to the hospital. I asked where the mother was and the father told me he had divorced her.

In some Middle Eastern countries men can divorce any one of their four wives by simply saying "I divorce you" three times, without any need to justify his actions. In this case, the father felt more than justified in getting rid of his "genetically-flawed" wife, without any consideration of her feelings nor the resulting emotional trauma to her son. From that moment on I decided I would no longer participate in this barbaric practice of eugenics. Islam, if anything, teaches its followers to accept Allah's will and this includes all the genetic diseases that abound there due to the high incidence of consanguinity resulting from the marriage of first and second cousins. Instead, I referred these cases to genetic counselors who, hopefully, would address more effectively the ethical and moral aspects of having a child affected with DMD.

Other neuromuscular disorders are more common in the Middle East than DMD. Congenital muscular dystrophy or sarcoglycanopathies, as well as spinal muscular atrophy (SMA) or Werdnig-Hoffman disease, were regularly seen in the clinic. Since these genetic disorders are inherited as autosomal recessive, both the mother and father contribute one defective gene each and one out four children are affected. In these cases, the father is equally responsible as his wife for transmission of the disease.

The plight of families who have children with DMD or SMA is a challenge to their dedication and resilience. The usually inexorable progression of weakness with little if any mental involvement can sear one's soul and even question our religious beliefs. Yet most parents I have seen exude generosity and understanding. They become examples to the community of the healing power of love, endless love.

McHenry LC Jr: *Garrison's History of Neurology.* Springfield, Ill.: Charles C. Thomas, Publisher, 1969.

33

AUTISM

Autism is a developmental disorder characterized by impaired social interaction, poor communication, and repetitive and stereotyped patterns of behavior, interest and activities. First described by Leo Kanner in 1943, autism has evolved in the past eighty years from an obscure and rare disorder to a more commonly recognized group of similar conditions encompassed under the vague "autism spectrum disorders" (ASD) and even less specific "pervasive developmental disorders" (PDD). Asperger syndrome refers to high-functioning autism with little if any impairment in social skills and speech.

According to the Centers for Disease Control and Prevention, the incidence of autism has been increasing and now affects 1 in 88 children. This increase is not explained by better recognition or overdiagnosis. Our clinics are now overwhelmed by referrals to evaluate neurologically autistic children. Except for the higher incidence of seizures, frequent history of early respiratory infections such as otitis media and global hypotonia, most referred children have no neurological abnormalities. Similarly, neurophysiological and neuroimaging studies, including brain wave recordings (EEG) and CT and MRI studies are mostly unremarkable.

Despite innumerable epidemiological, biochemical and genetic investigations, the etiology of autism remains elusive. The frustration many parents experience at the lack of explanations has resulted in incrimination of unlikely environmental factors such as mercury, vaccinations and contaminated foods. Vocal advocate groups have even proposed a conspiracy by the government to hide facts from the public about autism. Unfortunately, the more zealous proponents are targeted by individuals and groups without scruples promising remedies or even cures at considerable cost. These predators are consummate scam artists with uncanny abilities to convince and sell their products and services.

One of the many proposed but unproved hypotheses about autism is related to the frequent respiratory infections seen in these children during the first few years of life. The indiscriminate use of antibiotics may lead to overgrowth of the intestinal flora by yeast or fungal microorganisms, leading to the so-called "yeast factor" in autism.

Because of my interest in organic acidurias, I often sent to the laboratory urine samples for analysis on patients without a clear explanation for their symptoms, including autism. Several months later, the laboratory called and notified me that they had found an unusual pattern of organic acids in the urines of a group of children. A quick review of their medical records revealed the startling fact that all had a diagnosis of autism! Of particular interest were two brothers who had been extensively investigated elsewhere and found to have no etiological abnormalities. Both had a history of frequent bouts of otitis media treated with antibiotics during infancy.

The pattern of abnormal urine organic acids found was not associated with any known metabolic or organic acid disorder. Biochemical analysis of these metabolites using sophisticated gas chromatography and mass spectrometry (GC/MS) apparatus and techniques identified some of these as citramalic, tartaric, carboxycitric, 3-

oxoglutaric and phenylcarboxylic acids. Citramalic and tartaric were related to yeast metabolism and others were analogs of Krebs cycle metabolites. The urine samples obtained from twenty normal controls showed much lower concentrations of these metabolites.

An empirical trial of thiamine and pyridoxine in the two brothers resulted in symptomatic improvement. We decided then to run another empirical trial of antifungal treatment, using urine samples obtained before and after treatment for organic acid analysis. Mycostatin was used, as it is often prescribed for treatment in infants with monilial yeast infections because of its efficacy and safety. The preliminary results showed reduction in the concentrations of the yeast metabolites and parents observed symptomatic improvement in the children, often with clear advances in their language and social skills.

After publication of these preliminary findings, the "yeast hypothesis" began to gain in popularity and several laboratories across the country offered testing and treatment of autism at no small expense to the parents. Some of these laboratories approached us to be consultants and participate in the new "miraculous" treatment of autism. My answer was that these were only preliminary findings and that more data were necessary before we could recommend antifungal treatment for autistic children.

At this point I must mention the amazing improvement reported by parents of autistic children when treated with a new therapy—no matter what this may be. This is, undoubtedly, a placebo effect and no benefit is found in more strict and controlled studies. It is easy for parents and doctors to fall into this trap. Many years later, I wonder if this study should have been published or not. It was reviewed and approved for publication in a peer-reviewed chemistry journal. Our only intention was to instigate more research that might help elucidate the etiology of autism.

Throughout the years I have seen patients with incurable diseases treated with unconventional remedies: hyperbaric oxygen for cerebral palsy, stem cells for muscular dystrophy, massive doses of vitamins for intractable migraine, etc. Such unproven treatments are usually offered by unscrupulous individuals whose intent is to exploit desperate families. A few are convinced and really believe that they are helping these children—but not many. The advent of evidence-based medicine offers a more objective way to evaluate dubious therapeutic regimens.

Shaw W, Kassen E, Chaves E: Increased urinary excretion of analogs of Krebs cycle metabolites and arabinose in two brothers with autistic features. *Clinical Chemistry* 1995; 41: 1094-104.

34

STARTLE DISEASE

Hyperekplexia is a rare and interesting genetic disorder characterized by an exaggerated startle response to auditory or tactile stimulation. Although initially this was called hyperexplexia, an etymologist explained that the latter was an unacceptable combination of Greek and Latin and set the record straight with the more difficult to pronounce present designation.

Gilles de la Tourette, in his description of motor and vocal tics (which he called "tic convulsif", and now bears his eponym), discussed what he thought were allied conditions such as the "jumping men of Maine" who, as the name implies, would jump when suddenly startled, and "latah" in Malaya and "myriachit" in Siberia. There was also the curious phenomenon of cataplexy, seen in patients with narcolepsy when they laugh or cough loudly, resulting in them falling and unable to move. Even a breed of beagle dogs have a similar trait and when they bark loudly, will fall to the ground as if paralyzed by some internal process.

Unaware of the existence of hyperekplexia, I was much interested when a family was brought with several children who had this condition. The diagnosis was easily confirmed using the glabellar or nose tap sign, consisting of gently but briskly tapping the glabella (mid forehead) or nose tip with the index finger, resulting in a facial grimace, exaggerated eye blink and stiffening of the body. In normal persons, repetition of this maneuver attenuates or extinguishes the response by habituation. However, in patients with hyperekplexia the glabellar response is not attenuated, even if the individual already anticipates the repeated tapping of the glabella or nose tip.

Hyperekplexia would be nothing more than an interesting physiological phenomenon, except for the fact that the condition has a high mortality rate during infancy. In addition, there is also a high incidence of hypoxic-ischemic injury to the brain, resulting in cerebral palsy and other developmental handicaps. It is mainly inherited in an autosomal dominant manner, so that several family members are similarly involved.

Experienced nurses familiar with the disorder will alert the neonatalogist when they notice that one of the infants startles or jumps whenever there is a loud noise, as when a metallic object is dropped on the hard floor or a door slammed hard. The other infants merely squirm in their cribs, but the affected one has an exaggerated response to the auditory stimulus.

All of the information we had indicated that these infants were normal at birth but something occurred later on that put them at risk for brain injury. Eventually, it was discovered that as part of the exaggerated startle response, these infants suffered from laryngospasm (spasm of the larynx) and consequent interruption of the airway long enough or repeatedly enough to cause hypoxic-ischemic encephalopathy and later, cerebral palsy. We were able to document with serial brain wave tests (EEGs) that a normal brain electrical pattern at birth became abnormal shortly thereafter, showing abundant epileptiform discharges only a few days later. Unfortunately, we were not able to capture an episode of laryngospasm and the accompanying slowing of the brain waves to document the pathophysiology of brain injury in hyperekplexia—even though we tried using video-EEG.

Early identification of hyperekplexia is essential to prevent brain injury because treatment is simple and effective. Most patients with hyperekplexia respond well to administration of clonazepam, a benzodiazepine derivative. Small doses usually of 0.1 mg daily are sufficient to eliminate or control the exaggerated startle response. This treatment may be lifesaving and preventive for brain injury from hypoxia.

Hyperekplexia is caused by a defect in the *GLRA1* gene, which encodes the glycine receptor alpha-1 subunit. Glycine is an important amino acid neurotransmitter neuroinhibitor. Glycine receptors are more abundant in the brain stem and mediate important protective reflexes such as the blink response. Molecular genetic studies by Nadia Hejazi, one of our fellows training in child neurology, showed that some of our patients had a different genetic defect involving the beta-subunit of the glycine receptor and also that transmission was not autosomal dominant, but recessive. Unfortunately, these important findings were not published at the time.

After returning from the Middle East, I tried to identify hyperekplexia in suspected infants and children in the United States but was unable to find any. Tapping the tip of the nose or the glabella is such a simple test that it is worthwhile doing if a diagnosis of hyperekplexia may prevent brain injury or SIDS.

Hejazi NS, Chaves EC, Boumah C, et al: Linkage of hyperekplexia (HEK) in three Saudi families to chromosome 4q31.3 associated with glycine receptor beta subunit (GLRβ). *Neurology* 2001; 56 (Suppl 3): A132.

35

MIRACLE DOCTOR

According to Merriam-Webster's Collegiate Dictionary, a miracle is an extraordinary event manifesting divine intervention in human affairs. Most of us will transcend our lives without ever witnessing a miracle, although the second definition in my twenty-four-year-old dictionary includes an extremely outstanding or unusual event, thing, or accomplishment. The latter allows for a more vernacular use of the term and applies to less rare instances that, nevertheless, seem extraordinary and even at times difficult to believe as real or easily explained scientifically.

Miracles are easier to accept when based on spiritual or religious grounds. Faith is an important ingredient in the many miracles ascribed to spiritual leaders. Prayers and offerings abound in sacred locales throughout the world. In churches, basilicas, grottos, walls and tombs, pilgrims throng as earnest supplicants for favors to remedy their ailments. Many of these prayers are answered, as witnessed by the ecstatic faces of those who were paralyzed and now are able to walk, those who could not speak and now do so, and those who were blighted and are now cured.

The evangelists exemplified by Elmer Gantry, however, represent a different aspect of the business of miracles. Oral Roberts was a master of miracles and often surrounded by believers who witnessed the power of prayer and suggestion. Oral Roberts was so successful that he left a respected university as his legacy. But as a scientist, I have always been skeptical of miracles. Raised within a Catholic family who prayed the rosary and went to mass regularly, my religious indoctrination gradually faded as my scientific foundation was strengthened by the intrinsic truth of science, the veracity of Darwin's epochal writings, and realization that religions are man-made congregations that separate us instead of uniting us. Nevertheless, I have been inspired by a supernatural force upon entering the Notre Dame Cathedral in Paris on a Sunday morning and hearing the angelical choir soar into heaven, and as I vacillated in Salt Lake City in the ornate temple of the Church of Latter Day Saints. There was something sacred and inspiring in those places that I could not explain. Such a feeling, however, was lacking when I fulfilled my dream of visiting the site in Fatima, Portugal, where the three children saw the apparition of the Virgin Mary. The vast expanse failed to inspire me and all I could see was a massive tourist attraction that rivaled Disney World or Graceland.

Miracles are essential to the beatification and sanctification of extraordinary persons in the Catholic Church. Pope John Paul II decided to ease the requirements necessary to declare a person as a saint by reducing the number of miracles to two. During his papacy, more cardinals and saints were created than in any other period in the church's history. But how does the Catholic Church decide when a miracle can be ascribed to one of its devoted servants? What criteria are used? How many witnesses are required? How long does it take to substantiate an extraordinary event as a miracle?

The answers to these and other similar questions were sought by Jacalyn Duffin, a respected historian from

Queen's University in Toronto. Duffin obtained permission to examine the Vatican records on 1,400 miracles cited in canonizations between 1588 and 1999. Not surprisingly, the majority of these involved medical conditions. The amazing finding was that the church required a doctor's testimony as proof that a person had been cured, rather than more questionable and less reliable statements from church representatives. Thus, the church based the proof of a miracle on medical science and not on less scientific testimony.

Maria, a fifteen-year-old young lady, came to my clinic because she had an arachnoid cyst in her brain and needed a follow-up. Arachnoid cysts are congenital sacs of fluid lined by cells that form one of the three membranes that envelop the brain and represent benign lesions without complications unless these increase in size or compress more vital structures. As an example, I recently saw also a young man with an arachnoid cyst that occupied about *one third* of his brain space. He was asymptomatic, excellent student and his neurological examination was normal!

But back to Maria, our fifteen-year-old patient, who had been seen elsewhere and, therefore, I had not seen her lesion before. A routine MRI study was done and to our surprise, in addition to the arachnoid cyst which had not changed, there was a bright white (hyperintense), large lesion next to the tip of the right petrous (temporal) bone. The radiologist did not know what this lesion was and I sent the study to an expert neuroradiologist at a children's hospital elsewhere. The neuroradiologist reviewed the study and reported that, because of its appearance and location, this was a typical cholesterol granuloma, a lesion formed from epithelial cells that form keratin (horny layer) and other components related to the inner ear. Most of these lesions are removed surgically but I was reluctant to refer Maria to a neurosurgeon and advised the parents to better wait and repeat the MRI in six months. I also suspected the lesion had been there before and requested previous studies be sent to me for review. Sure enough, the lesion had been there before, although much smaller. Six months later the MRI was repeated and to our surprise (and delight), the cholesterol granuloma had disappeared! I had half-jokingly told the family that perhaps prayer might help, since I did not want any surgery at this time to remove the lesion. They were convinced that prayer had eradicated the lesion and called me from then on "the miracle doctor".

Duffin J. *Medical Miracles. Doctors, Saints, and Healing in the Modern World.* New York: Oxford University Press, 2009.

Stankovic KM, Eskandar E, El Khoury JB, et al. Case 2-2013: A 20-year-old man with recurrent ear pain, fever, and headache. *New England Journal of Medicine* 2013; 368: 267-77.

IV

OTHER MALADIES

36

LIFE AS AN INTERN

The internship program at Gorgas Hospital (then Ancon Hospital) in Panama began when William Gorgas wrote in 1905 to William Welch, the dean of American physicians at Johns Hopkins School of Medicine, asking him to recommend three recently graduated physicians for the posts of "internes" at a salary of $50 a month, room and board included.

The use of the words "interne" or "intern" and "resident" to categorize doctors in the early parts of their training probably has its origins from the hierarchical system of training physicians in French hospitals during the Nineteenth Century. An interne worked inside a hospital but lived outside the institution, while a resident was given the additional privileges of working and learning while living within the hospital. As expected, the position of resident was more prestigious than that of an intern.

Welch could only find one interne for Gorgas, and overqualified at that: Samuel Darling, already a pathologist with a solid background in bacteriology, who accepted the position only reluctantly. Darling would stay in Panama for the next ten years and in the process discover a new disease, histoplasmosis, solve the problem of malaria control by studying mosquitoes and identifying only one, *Anopheles albimanus*, as the one responsible for the transmission of malaria. This facilitated Gorgas' mandate to accomplish the sanitation of Panama and enabled the construction of the Panama Canal. The revised sanitation program made possible "species-specific control" aimed solely at eliminating the breeding habitat of this "urban" mosquito (as Gorgas called it) instead of covering the five-hundred square miles of the Canal Zone. Furthermore, Darling performed or supervised more than four thousand autopsies and published at least two hundred articles, case reports, and research studies on tropical diseases found in Panama.

I didn't know any of this at the time when I applied for a position as an intern at Gorgas Hospital upon completion of my medical studies in the United States in 1963. The internship was a rotating one and consisted of three-months' service each in Pediatrics, Surgery, Obstetrics/Gynecology and Internal Medicine. This required the intern to be "on call" every third day and night in the Emergency Room and accompany the ambulance when called to an accident site. In addition, any ship crossing the Panama Canal was entitled to free medical services. The sick crew either came to the hospital for evaluation or, in the case of a serious injury, the intern had to board the ship and assess the situation before the patient could be evacuated safely to the hospital.

In most situations, ship-call entailed the intern to board a tugboat with a large medical bag that housed everything one could possibly need to take care of any situation: from glass syringes, morphine vials, plaster rolls, to minor surgical instruments and sutures and needles, in addition to stethoscope, ophthalmoscope and reflex hammers. The only necessary help not included in the medical bag was an assistant! Most medical problems could be resolved by determining if the sick sailor needed hospitalization or not, and then evacuating the patient to Gorgas Hospital for further care.

The weather during the rainy season can suddenly turn nasty in tropical regions. On such a bad weather day, with strong winds and respectable swells, I answered a ship-call. The tugboat got as close as possible to the ship and when I was ready to climb aboard, all I saw was a rope ladder swinging wildly starboard. Despite the self-confidence of a young intern, not only did I fear falling and drowning in the Pacific Ocean, but trying to carry the large, heavy medical bag was tantamount, at least in my mind, to suicide. Despite leaving the medical bag behind, I tried to negotiate the moving rope strands with my hands and feet, avoiding looking down at the beckoning, merciless swells. The rest of the events of what happened on board the ship or what the medical problem was on that day, I don't have any clear recollection. I do remember, though, a great sense of relief when I placed my feet back on solid ground.

Ambulance calls were, for the most part, also quite mundane: car accidents required extrication of the victims from the twisted vehicles and then letting the orthopedists assume their care. However, I will never forget one fateful day that would appear in the cover of *Life* magazine: January 29, 1964.

On that unforgettable day, I was on duty in the Emergency Room at Gorgas Hospital, when a call came from the Tivoli Hotel that several wounded American soldiers needed medical attention. Wounded American soldiers in Panama? What was going on? The events had unfolded quietly but quickly escalated to a major confrontation between Panamanian citizens and American soldiers. Since the occupation of the Canal Zone by the Americans for the purpose of building the Panama Canal, Panamanians had resented the American presence in their territory and blamed the infamous Hay-Buneau-Varilla treaty as an affront to their sovereignty. The Canal Zone represented an American enclave, with its own police force, rules and regulations.

Racial discrimination in the Canal Zone not only targeted blacks but Panamanians as well. The discrimination included all employees of the Isthmian Canal Zone Commission, who were divided into two groups: the "gold roll" employees, who were American citizens and held the main administrative positions, and the "silver roll" employees, who were mainly African-Caribbean laborers brought from Jamaica, Barbados, Martinique and other Caribbean islands, and local Panamanians. The "gold roll" employees were paid in U.S. gold dollars, while the "silver roll" laborers were paid in Colombian pesos, roughly half of the equivalent pay. Up to the time I worked as an intern in the Canal Zone and for many years after, racial discrimination was pervasive everywhere in the Canal Zone: in the distribution of housing to employees, the commissary privileges, rest rooms, YMCA, etc. These pervading conditions only helped to kindle the resentment that most Panamanians had for the occupants of the Canal Zone.

A group of high-school students from the Instituto Nacional, located only a few blocks from the Fourth of July Avenue that divided the Canal Zone from the City of Panama, decided to march towards Balboa High School and raise the Panamanian flag alongside the flag of the United States. This was a peaceful march and, according to the treaty, both flags should fly together in the Canal Zone. Despite close monitoring of the situation by the Canal Zone police, the opposing student groups escalated from verbal to physical interchanges. That evening, snipers occupied the Pan American building on the Fourth of July Avenue and started shooting across to the Canal Zone. Aware that the Canal Zone police was insufficient to handle the situation, the U.S. Army was called to intervene. American soldiers were positioned strategically around the nearby Tivoli Hotel with strict orders not to shoot at civilians.

Close to midnight, I boarded the white Cadillac ambulance to pick up the wounded soldiers at the Tivoli Hotel. The ambulance driver unwittingly parked the white vehicle in front of the hotel and as I, dressed also in white, picked up my medical bag and emerged from the ambulance, heard shots and the wheezing sound of bullets over my head. Realizing the grave danger we were in, I dived back into the ambulance and shouted for the driver to get out of there immediately! From the back of the hotel, we then crawled and picked three soldiers wounded mainly in the legs with small firearms. By this time the radio and television were reporting the escalating crisis. The student demonstration had exploded into a national confrontation and the rest of the world watched with interest this battle between David and Goliath.

The next morning I was called to pick up a wounded policeman who had been hit in the head with a rock thrown by one of the Panamanian nationalists. As the ambulance descended from Ancon Hill to the Balboa Police Station, a large group of Panamanian students brandishing rocks and sticks stood menacingly, blocking our way. A young man, who appeared to be the leader, suddenly raised his hand and signaled for us to proceed peacefully. I remember distinctly our mutual eye contact and know that our fate was decided in that instant, for an attack by a horde of patriotic young men can quickly lead to disaster. I don't know who the student was, but I am sure I owe my life to his sense of respect and decency toward a young intern and his ambulance.

No one knows exactly the human toll from the January uprising. Official numbers from the Canal Zone

authorities reported four dead American soldiers, while
Panamanian reports vary but a reasonable number is
estimated as twenty-one deaths. The first victim and
considered a martyr, was Ascanio Arosemena, who was
killed by a stray bullet when he was trying to help an
injured citizen. The others who died are enshrined in a
monument in Panama City and the name of Fourth of July
Avenue has been changed to Avenue of the Martyrs.

During the conflagration, the Canal Zone was
closed to traffic and my wife and children, who were
visiting relatives in Panama City, were unable to return to
our home in Ancon Hill close to the hospital, until one
week later, when arrangements were made for us to meet at
a checkpoint near Curundu in the Canal Zone. Our
daughter, Maria, was born two days later.

An intern is like a foot soldier, ready to take orders
and to be on the firing line whenever necessary. Tired from
long working hours and lack of sleep, an intern is fueled
mainly by adrenaline and coffee to meet the demands that
come with the job. At the end of the grueling year, the only
rewards are the satisfaction of having completed this
archaic requirement and a small piece of paper attesting to
satisfactory completion of the internship. This certificate,
now yellowed by time and abandoned among other
certificates received from residencies, fellowships and
board examinations through the years, is the only one
which deserves a small footnote: *survived two life-
threatening experiences as an intern.*

Biesanz J: Race relations in the Canal Zone. *Phylon* 1950; 11:
23-30.

37

HAIR BIOPSIES

Hair may reflect not only ethnic characteristics of an individual, but also health status, including nutritional balance. Among developing countries where children suffer caloric and protein deprivation, hair may reflect these deficiencies. Kwashiorkor is an example of severe protein-calorie deficiency manifested by swelling (edema) due to hypoalbuminemia, skin lesions related to hypovitaminosis, and changes in hair color because of low tyrosine, a component of hair pigmentation. During alternate periods of insufficient protein intake intermixed with good nutrition, hair reflects these changes as the "flag sign", in which the hair color alternatively lightens and darkens, respectively, and these appear as stripes. Other examples of hair abnormalities are the coarse hair seen hypothyroidism and other endocrinopathies.

Early on, my interest in the microscopic examination of hair was motivated by the thought that this was an easily accessible sample which might provide clues to underlying disorders. Most of the time mothers had no objection when I asked permission to take a few strands of hair for examination. Using my trusted Swiss Army knife, this was a simple, painless procedure. The hair strands were placed on a glass slide and then covered with clear Scotch tape, for review later in the laboratory. After looking at hundreds of these, I concluded early on that "hair biopsies" yielded very little, if any, useful diagnostic information.

Nevertheless, there are some rare but interesting hair morphological variations in certain congenital metabolic disorders (inborn errors of metabolism). Kinky-hair disease, first described by John Menkes, is one of these. Examination of the hair under low-power magnification shows hair shafts that are kinked at right angles (*pili torti*) and hence the descriptive name of the disease, which is also known as Menkes' disease. This turned out to be a metabolic disorder due to lack of copper-transporting enzymes and treatment with supplemental copper may reverse the mental retardation and progressive course. Another metabolic disorder, argininosuccinic aciduria, is accompanied by hair shafts that seem to be broken and leave a tufted end that looks like a brush. This type of hair abnormality is called *trichorrhexis nodosa*, almost as complicated to pronounce as the name of the underlying amino acid disorder. Finally, there is a third type of hair abnormality, *monilethrix*, which is not specific for any disorder but reflects poor internal or external source of proteins and appears under the microscope as a progressive thinning of the hair shaft.

More recently, a child came to see us who had a peculiar type of hair abnormality. Not only was his hair thin, reddish and straight—almost standing on end and giving him the appearance of being frightened—but sparse as well. Lacking for a better term, other similar cases have been described as having "frizzy hair." Although it was thought initially that he might have *trichothiodystrophy*, microscopic examination of his hair with polarized light did not confirm the diagnosis.

Trichotillomania, or the pathological repeated pulling of hair from the scalp, is linked to compulsive behavior as seen in autism and pervasive developmental disorders. For years, when I was bored at administrative meetings, I pulled all the hairs I could find on my ears. Out of respect, I guess, no one mentioned that I had *trichotillomania*. I was born with absence of scalp hair in a small patch in my left temporal region. This is called *alopecia areata* and used to be a sign of syphilis. I was told by a dear aunt that this is where they put "extra brains" in my head. Finally, to complete this piece on relatively useless information about hair, the common English phrase "pulling my leg" is translated into Spanish as "pulling my hair" (*tomar el pelo*).

38

URINE ACIDS

Examination of the urine to detect diseases has been practiced by alchemists and physicians for centuries, if not millennia. Of all the body fluids available, it is the easiest to procure and examine. Color, density, odor and turbidity are some of the urine physical characteristics that may have diagnostic value. Furthermore, microscopic examination of the urine will reveal the presence or absence of red blood cells (hematuria), pus cells, crystals, casts and even certain parasites. Chemically, the urine will show glucose in diabetes, protein in kidney disease, uric acid crystals in gout, and ketones in acidosis. The acidity of the urine is also measured but is of little diagnostic value. The typical urinalysis or UA as it is known in the laboratory, consists of describing its appearance, pH (acidity), specific gravity (density), presence of glucose and protein, and results of microscopic examination for red and white blood cells.

The urine also contains products eliminated through the kidneys from the blood. These products are mostly end-products of metabolic cycles no longer useful to us but also represent substances such as drugs or toxic compounds which are eliminated after their neutralization by glucuronidation for easier transport through the glomerular membrane. Thus, the urine provides a source of information about glucose, protein and lipid (fat) metabolism, as well as evidence about exposure to extrinsic chemicals that enter our system either by design or accidentally.

One of the most sophisticated analytical tools available to chemists is gas liquid chromatography (GLC). A mixture of compounds is first separated by passing the sample through a column packed with a finely ground inert material such as silica. The silica is impregnated with a specific compound selected because of its known affinity for the group of metabolites of interest. An inert gas such as helium is passed through the column at a certain pressure to separate the admixture according to specified physico-chemical properties such as molecular weight, electronic charge, etc. A spectrophotometer at the end detects each compound and also measures its abundance or concentration.

A second and even more sophisticated apparatus, a mass spectrometer (MS), bombards each compound as it emerges from the GLC apparatus with highly-charged electrons, creating a group of component particles which resembles a "fingerprint" for each compound of interest. The merging of these two analytical technologies is known as gas chromatography/mass spectrometry (GC/MS). Before computers became common tools in the laboratory, this unique fingerprint or "mass spec" pattern for each compound had to be searched in paper databases until an exact match was found. Needless to say, the process took hours until computerized databases made easy work of this type of search. GC/MS could now be applied to more practical endeavors, such as identification of illegal drugs in athletes, toxic compounds in forensic medicine and, of particular interest to me, inborn errors of metabolism (IEM).

My first exposure to GLC was an antiquated apparatus that had been kept in good working condition during my research on lipids as a neurology resident. Packing the columns, extracting the body fluid of interest and interpreting the results obtained did not justify in my mind the time invested in this type of analysis. The coupling of mass spectrometry (MS) to gas chromatography (GC), however, converted this into a powerful analytical tool capable of identifying practically any compound of interest. The process of identification, however, still was time-consuming until databases became computerized. Hewlett-Packard® was one of the innovators of GC/MS technology and eventually the cost became less prohibitive.

My first complete and modern GC/MS Hewlett-Packard® apparatus was acquired while I worked at Eastern Virginia Medical School in Norfolk, Virginia. After my clinical obligations in the clinic and hospital seeing patients were met, I then spent several hours in the laboratory using GC/MS to study several challenging projects. First of all, samples from patients were analyzed looking for inborn errors of metabolism. One evening, as I was looking at the results obtained that day, the excitement of our first positive analysis emerged. The characteristic and diagnostic pattern of glutaric aciduria was unmistakable. I called the referring doctor and proudly gave him the diagnosis.

One of the first research projects involved the study of newborns with sepsis. Sepsis is a diagnosis made frequently in the newborn nursery when an infant is sick but no good explanation is found to explain it. Cultures of blood, urine and cerebrospinal fluid are, most of the time, negative. My thinking was that such a population must harbor some unidentified inborn errors of metabolism and a protocol was devised to collect and analyze urine samples from these sick infants in my laboratory. After several years of processing these samples, not a single case of IEM was identified, due to the low incidence of these rare disorders, ranging from 1:10,000 to 1:100,000 newborns. Even if our nursery had five hundred births per year, it would take a long time to come across one single case of IEM. Yet this was a good learning experience, as I learned to readily identify urine abnormalities in infants such as the presence of lactic acid, antibiotics and other medications given to sick newborns.

A second project was the analysis of body fluids, including urine and vitreous humor (obtained post-mortem), for organic acids in sudden infant death syndrome (SIDS) victims. With the cooperation of the local medical examiner, a number of samples were obtained from twenty-five SIDS victims and analyzed by GC/MS. Again, none were diagnostic for an IEM, probably for the same reason: an insufficient number of patients.

These laborious studies were, unfortunately, mostly unproductive and, therefore, did not merit full-length publications. Some appeared in abstract form and were presented at neurological meetings. Even though my investigations using GC/MS gave poor results, the time spent in the laboratory gave me a great deal of satisfaction. Not all research results in groundbreaking discoveries. I also worked alone, without collaboration from others who might have given me new ideas or stimulated different avenues of research. Many great discoveries are not only the result of hard work but also of serendipity. Serendipity, unfortunately, was not a close ally in my laboratory.

Chaves-Carballo E: Metabolic encephalopathies and sudden infant death syndrome. *Annals of Neurology* 1994: 36: 297.

Chaves-Carballo E: Rett's syndrome: urine organic acid abnormalities. *Annals of Neurology* 1987; 22: 442.

Chaves-Carballo E: Glutaric aciduria type I responsive to riboflavin. *Neurology* 1988; 38 (Suppl 1): 293.

Chaves-Carballo E: Fumaric aciduria (FA): A mitochondrial encephalopathy associated with sudden infant death syndrome. *Neurology* 1989; 39 (Suppl 1): 190.

39

FAMILIAR FOOTSTEPS

The concept of a sleuth and astute observer, enshrined by Sir Arthur Conan Doyle (1859-1930) in the character of Sherlock Holmes, may have originated on the observational skills of two medical doctors: Joseph Bell and Henry Littlejohn.

Physicians are trained early in the required skills of observation, palpation, percussion and auscultation to arrive at a correct diagnosis. These skills are essential in the recognition of presenting signs of certain diseases (the butterfly rash in lupus, slapped appearance in scarlatina, acneform lesions in tuberous sclerosis—to name only a few diagnostic facial characteristics). The human brain contains about twenty billion neurons and seventy trillion synapses or connections, acting as a most sophisticated computer to process information. A physician gathers the information from the detailed history and physical examination, feeds it to the brain and expects an answer after processing the information that will help arrive at a diagnosis.

The recognition of familiar faces is one of the earliest cognitive skills developed in infancy, possibly even after only a few weeks of life. The loss of this skill, usually later in life from strokes, is called *prosopagnosia*. Oliver Sacks popularized this distressing neurological condition in his book, *The Man Who Mistook his Wife for a Hat*. Imagine daily life without the ability to recognize familiar faces. Even when looking at a mirror, we would not be able to identify our own image!

Akin to the identification of others by looking at the face, posture is also a unique attribute to each one of us and sometimes we are able to identify a person from behind by the posture: the inclination of the head, position of the shoulders, bending angle of the back, etc. Each person is unique in the sum of all these physical attributes. Our identification skills, though, may not be infallible, as when we recognize our error and apologize, "I am so sorry, but I thought you were…."

From the time an infant is delivered and his or her feet are stained with ink to mark his footprints (instead of fingerprints) for identification, using mainly the creases and wrinkles which are relatively unique to each, to later on when independent gait is attained, to the slow and methodical placement of the feet when we reach an older age, feet are as much a part of our physiognomy as our faces are.

I used to think that a newborn infant's feet mainly reflected their position in utero. That is, the deviation of the feet and toes was the result of the small compartment and that the appearance of the feet later on depended on mechanical forces during fetal development. This idea I discarded many years ago in favor of the genetic or inherited explanation. Each one of us is the result of traits inherited from our parents. The way we look, the way we talk, the way we walk and even the way we think and reason, are mostly the result of inherited traits. We may group these traits into families, nationalities and even ethnic groups.

For many years, I have closely observed children's feet. Some are wide and some are thin; some are short and some are long; some have high arches and others have flat feet (*pes planus*); some are pigeon-toed (*metatarsus adductus*) and some are not. But in every case, children's feet resemble their parents' feet. Not only the feet themselves, but how they function—that is, how they walk. The manner in which an individual places the foot on the ground, the angle of deviation of the foot from the midline, the position of the ankle (*varus* or *valgus*) with regard to the foot, etc. These are all, for the most part, inherited traits. But what if each parent has widely different traits? Which one predominates? Most of the time, I think, the child represents a combination of the two.

To test this hypothesis, or merely to learn how to apply it, just for fun, from now on observe closely those walking ahead of you. Look at their feet and try to note any resemblance in their gaits. Father and son are easily identified by their gait similarities, while father and mother differ substantially. Brothers and sisters are also quite similar among themselves and different from cousins and friends-at-large. Different ages have little to do with this, as grandparents also resemble the way their grandchildren walk, or vice versa. The way we walk is mainly a genetic trait, although it can be altered by disease or accidents. It is almost impossible for any of us to change this at will. Although once I saw a mime in Key West who had the uncanny ability to imitate any person who walked by, causing observers to laugh at the expense of the victim, who was unaware of this consummate imitator. Of all the great imitators, none more skilled than Rich Little, who had almost a hundred characters he imitated—not only in the way they talked, but walked and gestured as well. Some characters are easier to imitate than others: Charlie Chaplin, Jack Benny, James Cagney, John Wayne and, of course, Elvis.

40

PREGNANT FROGS

One of the most difficult tests I learned to do when I worked at a university hospital as a laboratory technician was the urine pregnancy test. Fifty years ago, this was not done by simply impregnating a stick with urine and observing the telltale change in color. The pregnancy test then required the use of frogs and, more specifically, the toad *Bufo americanus.*

The toads were housed in a wire-cage and, almost as a reflex, as soon as this was opened, they jumped and chasing a toad all over the laboratory floor was part of the rite. I found out that the best practice was to grab the toads by their hind legs and then suspend them upside down for a better grip. The next step consisted of injecting under the skin a couple of milliliters of concentrated urine from the patient. After a few hours, the toad's cloaca (posterior opening) was catheterized using a small glass capillary tube and the toad's urine than placed on a glass side for microscopic examination, looking for frog sperm, presumably stimulated by the excess hormones present in the urine. Performing the test was actually fun, but time-consuming and sometimes there were more urgent requests such as a stat blood sugar or a type-and-cross match for blood from the Emergency Room.

I have had little sympathy for frogs or toads throughout my life. As a child I was told that some had poison on their skin and, therefore, should not touch them (which was fine with me). The distinction between a frog and a toad, in my mind, was based mainly on the degree of ugliness. I will eat frog legs, but in doing so try not to think about the *New Yorker* cartoon showing a row of frogs coming out in wheelchairs from a restaurant serving frog legs. Tennessee Ernie Ford, in one of the early programs in black-and-white television, would sooner or later say, "looked bug-eyed like a stepped-on toad," and sent everybody in the audience laughing. One of my professors would come out with a similar (he was also from Tennessee) saying, "bright-eyed and bushy-tailed" when referring to a hyperactive child.

One of the most ingratiating frogs, though, is the red-eyed green frog (*Agalychnis callidrys*) found in Costa Rica. Measuring less than three inches in length, it resembles the Kermit character from the Muppets and would be a popular tourism ambassador. Other frogs in Costa Rica are the colorful dart-poison frogs of the genus *Dendrobates*. The latter exhibit *aposematism*, the use of bright red and yellow colors to warn predators of their unpalatable toxicity. Many of these small amphibians are in danger of extinction as a result of *chytridiomycosis*, a fungal infection that coats their permeable skin and prevents proper oxygenation of their tissues.

One of my favorite grandchildren's photographs shows one of them holding a bullfrog that seems longer than he is tall, with a triumphant grin on his face (my grandson—not the frog). I suppose this is a rite every boy has to pass at a certain age. When we first saw this huge frog, he looked at it and started to walk away, when I suddenly yelled, "Grab it!" His hesitation must have lasted only a few milliseconds because before I knew it, he had snatched the amphibian before he could leap to safety and then paraded his trophy to the rest of our family. An experience like that may become a treasured memory in a grandfather's mind, displacing the antics associated with frog pregnancy tests many years before.

41

LIBRARIES AND BOOKS

The *Biblioteca Nacional* in San José, Costa Rica, was a venerable structure located only two blocks away from the *Avenida Central*, the main thoroughfare in the city. Separated by thick stone walls from the outside noise created by humans and motor vehicles, the reading room was as silent as any cathedral during high mass.

Communication was mediated mainly by whispering and any sound above the allowed decibels brought swiftly reprimanding stern gazes from the proverbial librarian with thick glasses. Our forays into this temple of learning were limited to the weekly assignments given to us by our admired and respected Spanish teacher, Esther de Mézerville. She expected the students to recite in front of the class on the following week, the biography of a prominent Spanish or Latin American literature giant. The library usually had, as if anticipating our needs, a typewritten biography consisting of three to five pages representing the second or third carbon copy of the original on onionskin, fragile paper. Legibility and integrity were compromised by repeated use by students over the years. Xerox® had not invented the copy machine yet and the biography was copied by hand in our *cuadernos* or notebooks. After an hour or so, we left the library for a quick stroll and then home. The copied biography would then be committed to memory by repeating again and again until we know we could easily recite it next week if were unlucky enough to be chosen by the teacher to stand in front of the class and regurgitate our notes. If we learned little about famous authors, this exercise did train us to speak in front of an audience, although one student could not overcome the challenge of public speaking and she would cry inconsolably until the teacher allowed her to sit down again.

My reverence for libraries and books developed much later in college and became a magnificent obsession in medical school and residency training centers. The first journal I subscribed to was the *New England Journal of Medicine* and the first bound volume dated 1964 still occupies the first stall in my bookshelves. For years I read every article in this venerable weekly journal and were it not for my reluctance to openly participate at conferences, I would have surprised the professors with my fund of general medical knowledge. My subscription to this journal has remained uninterrupted for over fifty years, although now I am more selective and only read those articles that pique my interest.

Before the days of digitized and computerized databases, the library was the only place where needed references could be found. This required an arduous review of the *Index Medicus* published by the National Library of Medicine in thick monthly volumes that lined shelves or above long tables in the center of the library. A review of the literature signified a commitment of time that could last months or even years, since every volume had to be searched for publications pertaining to the subject of interest and "complete" meant really complete, at times searching for cross-references quoted in other languages, including French, Italian, German, Russian and even Hungarian or Romanian. Use of bilingual dictionaries to decipher the international publication meant additional weeks of work.

My first attempt at such a review of the literature concerned a case of Üllrich-Turner syndrome in a male (probably a case of unrecognized Noonan syndrome). The review of the literature took about a year and many evenings pouring over collections of bound journals. Fortunately, the medical center had one of the most complete journal collections in the world and this facilitated the search for obscure references. Report of the index case and review of the literature were published in the *Mayo Clinic Proceedings* and many requests for reprints were received and answered. The library became for me a second home and a sanctuary for reading, writing and meditating about medicine.

Another refuge for me during my years in Panama (1967-1972) was the medical library at Gorgas Hospital in the Canal Zone. Mrs. Virginia Ewing Stich, the medical librarian, had saved everything related to the medical history of the isthmus of Panama, especially the sanitation of Panama by William Gorgas. Gorgas had eliminated yellow fever and controlled malaria sufficiently in Panama so that the American enterprise to build an interoceanic canal would not suffer the same fate that the French and Ferdinand de Lesseps (1805-1894), the builder of the Suez Canal, had experienced in Panama. Her task was not an easy one, since each new hospital director wanted to take home as souvenirs important documents that recorded the medical history of Panama. Mrs. Stich was an admirer of Samuel Taylor Darling, whom she remembered walking daily to the hospital from his home, tall and handsome, with his red hair and goatee, immersed in his own thoughts as many other geniuses have done in the past.

Darling had learned pathology in Baltimore after graduating first in his 1903 class at the Baltimore College of Physicians & Surgeons (now University of Maryland School of Medicine). Two days after his marriage to Nannyrle Llewellyn, a nursing student from Virginia, he accepted an offer to join Gorgas in Panama as an "interne," a job for which he was overqualified. Nevertheless, he was convinced by Henry Carter, hospital director, that this was a great opportunity and that, once he proved himself, he would be promptly promoted. The salary as an intern was $50 a month and, according to the rule of the Canal Zone, he was entitled to only one square foot per dollar for his housing. Needless to say, his wife did not join him until six months later, when his salary was substantially increased.

But Darling had little interest in money or social standing. He was a dedicated pathologist and spent most of his time studying tropical disease and performing autopsies, of which he did himself or supervised more than four thousand during his ten-year stay in Panama. Scarcely one year after his arrival in Panama, on December 7, 1905, Darling did an autopsy on a 27-year-old Martiniquan and after completing the gross examination, concluded that the man had died of tuberculosis. However, later on that same day, he returned to the laboratory to examine the slides he had made of the lesions in the lungs and other organs. To his delight, he found myriad of microorganisms he had never seen before and called these *Histoplasma capsulatum* on the incorrect assumption that these were a protozoan (later proved to be a fungus). Darling had just discovered the first case of histoplasmosis in the world. Within six months, he would encounter the same microorganism in two more cases and reported these in several articles published in respected medical journals.

The discovery of histoplasmosis would have sufficed to assure Darling a prominent place in the pantheon of medical discoveries. But he was tireless and before he left Panama at the time of the completion of the canal, he had authored more than two hundred publications on tropical diseases and other subjects that attracted his interest. Among his more important contributions was his monograph on malaria, *Studies on Malaria*, which established his reputation as a malariologist and converted his laboratory into a mecca for pathologists and parasitologists from all over the world, who wanted to meet and learn from this extraordinary scientist.

After leaving Panama, Darling joined the Rockefeller Foundation and spent several years in Sumatra, Ceylon (Sri Lanka), Malaya and other exotic places, where he was content analyzing fecal samples for intestinal parasites. His reports on hookworm evidence his brilliant investigations and showed the world the need for better control of these diseases. Unfortunately, Darling died in 1924 in a motorcar accident while returning to Beirut as a member of the Malaria Commission of the League of Nations. He had been elected president of the American Society of Tropical Medicine and invited to address the Royal Society of Tropical Medicine and Hygiene (along with Gorgas) in London but his untimely death prevented him from enjoying these singular honors.

Mrs. Stitch and I talked frequently about Darling and his accomplishments. We both agreed that Darling had been "the forgotten man" and that we should do something to keep his memory alive. The idea came but took a long time to fulfill, thanks to petty squabbles with administrators. However, on October 27, 1972, the medical library at Gorgas Hospital was officially named the

"Samuel Taylor Darling Memorial Library" and a bronze plaque placed that read:

Samuel Taylor Darling Memorial Library
In Recognition of his Contributions
To Medical Knowledge
Chief of Laboratories—Ancon Hospital 1905-1915
Physician, Pathologist and Parasitologist
1872-1925

After retirement from her position as librarian at Gorgas Hospital and concerned about her advancing age, Mrs. Stich approached me about writing a medical history of the Canal Zone. Although the idea was attractive to me, I did not want to commit to something I may have not been able to complete. In one of my last visits to Mrs. Stich's home in New Orleans, she proudly gave me two valuable items in her possession: 1) a complete collection of the *Proceedings of the Canal Zone Medical Association* spanning the years 1908 to 1927; and 2) the other and even more valuable document was Darling's original autopsy record of his first case of histoplasmosis. Darling's bold, left-handed strokes and the ravages of time and humidity had conspired against this document. Fortunately, a visiting American admirer of Darling's work took it back to the United States and had it restored as much as was possible, applying similar preservation techniques as used for the Dead Sea scrolls.

I was unable to find the time necessary to honor Mrs. Stich's expectations of me. I had slowly collected much information and received a grant-in-aid by the Rockefeller Foundation to visit their archives in North Tarrytown, New York, for a week. Thanks to the admirable record keeping policies of the Rockefeller Foundation,

Darling's life and activities during his years in the Far East could be reconstructed and solidified in a coherent manner. The poor record keeping of the Isthmian Canal Commission, however, resulted in the loss of most of Darling's personal correspondence and, hence, this could not be pieced together with any historical validity, except from what could be gleaned from his own publications.

Finally, after retirement from active practice in 2002, I was able to concentrate on my unfinished business. If I had known at the beginning how much time and effort would be required to write a book about Darling's life and work, I may have been easily dissuaded to concentrate my efforts on something else. But Mrs. Stich's inspiration kept me at work and six years later, Darling's biographical work appeared in print. *Samuel Taylor Darling. Parasites, Pathology and Philanthropy* was published in the U.K. in 2007, and consisted of 260 pages and more than 500 references. The book's sales did not reach a hundred copies, so that I received not one cent from its publication. However, I have seldom been more proud of anything I have done in the past. I know Mrs. Stich is smiling at me from somewhere up there, where generous souls dwell after they have sowed the seeds that inspire the rest of us.

Chaves-Carballo E: *The Tropical World of Samuel Taylor Darling. Parasites, Pathology and Philanthropy.* Brighton, U.K.: Sussex Academic Press, 2007.

42

MEDICAL WRITING

One of the benefits of retirement is more time available to do things we wanted to do but found little time for before. For me, this was predominantly reading and writing. Being proficient in both English and Spanish, I have benefited from both the beauty of Latin languages and the precision of Anglo-Saxon lexicography.

Someone once said that Spanish was the language to speak to God, Italian the language to speak to women, French the language to speak to men and German the language to speak to horses. In today's world, the two most representative languages are Spanish and English. Spanish is romantic and the beauty of poetry by Pablo Neruda is, in my opinion, superior to Shakespeare's sonnets. Poetry is still much alive in the Spanish-speaking world, while it languishes in obscurity in the English realm. On the other hand, English is scientific, descriptive, precise and unequaled in the world as the language of choice. Spanish has adopted many English words and today's youth speak a curious mixture called "Spanglish".

A medical history in Spanish is presented by the student or resident in ornate and flowery phrases, while in English there is an economy of words and details are exact with little if any modifiers. I regularly read a Spanish neurological journal, *Revista de Neurología*, and still marvel at the elegance of a routine case presentation.

Among my favorite medical writers are Macdonald Critchley, Oliver Sacks, Richard Selzer and Atul Gawande. Each one writes in English but differently in the sense that each inspires the reader using different techniques. Macdonald Critchley, an English neurologist, in his *The Divine Banquet of the Brain* and other essays describes eloquently the grandiosity of neurology and its pioneers. Oliver Sacks, on the other hand, is less inspiring but more interesting as he describes in detail unusual patients with challenging neurological problems. Richard Selzer is more philosophical and his books have memorable cases such as that of Imelda, the young Filipino girl, on whom he repaired a cleft lip post-mortem so her family could see how beautiful she was when she entered heaven. Atul Gawande is more practical and in *Complications* exposes modern medicine's fallacies and in the *New Yorker* essay "Big Med" compares the inefficiency of modern hospitals with the finely honed operation of a successful restaurant franchise.

Medical writing is difficult. Peer-reviewed journals are now more selective and demanding. Publishing articles on medical history, as I do, becomes even more problematic, since only a few journals remain dedicated to this discipline. Some years ago, I went to a national meeting of a society for medical historians. This was one of the most boring meetings I remember ever attending! Each presentation was read as an essay and lost the spontaneity and simple description of interesting facts. The word *historiography* has now become the popular currency, although I still don't fully understand its meaning. I vowed not to attend another history of medicine meeting. I dislike pomposity and obscure ideas.

Editors and publishers have become the ultimate arbiters of what is published and what is not. Why not let the readers decide what is good and what is bad? Hopefully, e-books, independent and self-publishing presses will break this monopoly that threatens to extinguish good medical writing and topple demanding and unreasonable editors from their pedestals.

43

EXPERT WITNESS

An expert witness is an individual recognized as an expert in his or her chosen field and retained by the plaintiff or the defendant to defend his or her position in court.

Lawyers find expert witnesses by scanning lists of leaders in academic positions who have demonstrated proficiency in publications such as journal articles or books that attest to their expertise in certain subjects. Also important is the experience of the expert witness in previous cases demonstrating confidence, solid knowledge and ability to withstand jarring questions and statements from opposing attorneys questioning credentials, honesty and professionalism. Like in so many other endeavors, practice makes perfect and the novice expert witness is more likely to be rattled and become angry than a seasoned older professor who has dealt with this process many times before.

The predictable court sessions in television series and suspenseful dramatizations narrated by John Grisham do not depict, in my opinion, accurately what happens in real life. An expert witness is first contacted by an attorney who wants to know if this particular case has any merit. A brief description by telephone may be sufficient to determine that the attorney's client does not have a case and further action would be futile. More often than not, the decision cannot be made until all medical records and previous testimonies are reviewed by the expert witness. The delivery by U.P.S.® or Federal Express® of several boxes of three-ring binders, each containing meticulously partitioned subjects, means several days and many hours reading and evaluating each document. The expert witness is paid for this activity by the hour at a pre-determined rate, just as the lawyers have also established for themselves. The most expensive expert witnesses at the time were usually neurosurgeons who received remuneration of at least $500 an hour.

After the expert witness has reviewed all the material received about the case in question, a meeting is arranged with the interested attorney to discuss the details of the case and formulate a strategic plan for its defense. Although this initial encounter may sound informal, the expert witness may be asked to disclose everything that was discussed during the session and, therefore, has to be cautious of any frivolous comments or opinions that may require disclosure by request of the opposing legal team. Needless to say, copious notes may be taken and these are also subject to disclosure if the other side wants to examine them.

For a professional who has escalated the hierarchy of academic advancement, from instructor to assistant professor to associate professor to full professor, facing an aggressive adversary who starts by questioning your personal integrity or professional credentials can be quite unnerving. Did you fail your board examination or did you pass the first time? Have you ever been denied a license to practice medicine? Have you ever received a ticket for driving under the influence (DUI)? These are initial questions designed to gauge your patience and ability to respond under stress. To take any of these as a personal affront is to invite disaster and will earn a wry smile from your executioner. You are now doomed as an expert witness.

The opposing lawyer now is ready to tackle the question if you are or are not a credible expert witness. The list of publications in your curriculum vitae (CV) must have support for your claim of expert knowledge. Each publication may have been carefully read and its merits questioned. Did you use controls? Did you support your conclusions by sound statistical analysis? Who really did the work and who wrote the paper or book? How many cases have you actually seen before of this disease? Again, be cool and not let anything ruffle your feathers. Above all, never lie or hesitate. Any sign of weakness may be and *will be* held against you.

At this point, the next item in the agenda is to show that you are "a hired gun" (which you are anyway) by demonstrating that most of your previous actions as an expert witness have been for the defense of a fellow physician and not for the injured patient. This will cast a shadow on your objectivity and uncover your bias that the doctor is always right and the patient's complaint has no merit. You must then have a well-balanced list of cases to prove your willingness to defend whoever is right, no matter if doctor or patient.

These preliminary sessions are usually held at one of the attorney's plush conference rooms, attended by several legal advisers from both camps, as well as a stenographer who transcribes every word for the record. A coffee or rest room break is called about every hour or the questioning party may ask if the proceedings may continue uninterrupted. These breaks are also used for the benefit of the opposing parties, who may decide to change or strengthen their strategy based on what has transpired already.

The most difficult part of the meeting comes next. The opposing lawyer is given the courtesy of questioning the expert witness first. The assailant has incredible anamnestic memory and will try to trick you by testing your knowledge of the facts and verify your thoroughness when reviewing the voluminous records. If you are able to pass successfully the factual examination, then the lawyer elevates his game to the next level by asking either succinct questions that demand only a monosyllabic answer: "yes" or "no," or open-ended questions thrown like a fishing lure to tempt you to bite and fall into the hands of the opposition. One of the most important rules the expert witness has to learn early in the game is not to give any more information than necessary; less than necessary is even better. The expert witness has the advantage of having more medical knowledge and experience than the legal experts. If used with caution, this advantage may very well win the case for your side.

Another strategy employed by the opposing lawyer is to ask a question that has more than one part, thus requiring more than one answer. The expert witness at this point may be close to exhaustion, both physically and mentally, and show exasperation or anger. A seasoned expert witness will calmly reply, "Your question, sir, has one or more parts. Please rephrase this so that I can answer one at a time." Still another modus operandi is to ask leading questions, at times subtle enough that you may not perceive them as such. Always listen to your counselor when he or she promptly interjects, "Objection! The examiner is leading the witness." Do not think you can outsmart the examiner on your own, but wisely refrain from answering and regretting your response.

Finally, an expert witness has to learn how to use deftly a couple of legal statements. The use of these two concluding phrases resembles the culminating moment when a wife asks her husband, or a culinary expert seeks a final opinion about the meat loaf or steak tartare. The answer determines the future course of action and whether the case will be taken to court or settled out of court—the latter to everyone's advantage. The first of these statements is usually posed as a question: "Doctor, in your opinion, is it more likely than not, that the client suffered an injury as a result of the doctor's negligence?" Here the modifying phrase "more likely than not" is a quantitative assessment indicating that the probability is more than 50 percent. The other question is more tenuous but has to be answered unequivocally as well: "Doctor, in your opinion, did the patient receive from the doctor (or hospital) treatment conforming to the standard of care?"   Again, these questions must be answered "yes" or "no." Any further elaboration or explanation by the expert witness will usually be curtailed promptly by the defense: "Doctor, just answer the question as 'yes' or 'no,' please!"

Should the attorneys be unable to "settle" or reach an agreement, the case may then go to court. This may entail months or even years before the final decision is made, a situation no one desires. Rarely, the defending client (usually a doctor) will not want to appear as compromising his or her reputation and refuses to settle, carrying on the proceedings all the way to the end. More than one doctor has found out about the futility of this posture and the exorbitant cost it entails.

Modesty aside, I have never "lost" a case in which I was an expert witness. This is not to say that I was smarter than the opposing lawyers—far from it. I was fortunate to select cases that had sufficient merit to justify my participation. The closest I came to losing was one case of hypoxic-ischemic encephalopathy in which I gave a written expert opinion that the child's disability was not caused by birth asphyxia, only to change my mind and reverse my previous position a couple of years later. This looked like an expert witness' nightmare and a win-win situation for the opposing attorneys.

This case illustrates how medicine is an evolving science and what may be considered to be the truth today may not be the same tomorrow. As a pediatric neurologist, I was taught that an infant who is born with low Apgar scores (a numbering system that gives a newborn infant a score from 0 to 10, indicating color, respiratory effort, heart rate, response to stimulation and muscle tone) had suffered from birth asphyxia and this was the cause of his or her cerebral palsy. However, in the 1970s, Karin Nelson, a pediatric neurologist working at NIH, studied a large cohort of fifty-eight thousand pregnant women who were followed prospectively throughout the pregnancy and the progeny until age seven years. Nelson, in collaboration with statistician Jonas Ellenberg, published three landmark articles that refuted the established notion that birth asphyxia was the main cause of cerebral palsy. The results of these epidemiological studies, known as the National Collaborative Perinatal Project (NCPP), concluded that birth asphyxia was not the cause of the majority of cases of cerebral palsy. A national collective groan was heard from the legal community who had made a comfortable living blaming obstetricians for children with spastic diplegia or spastic quadriplegia. Because of this important study published by Nelson and Ellenberg, I concluded that, in my opinion, the case I had reviewed had satisfied the standard of care and that it was more likely than not that the cerebral palsy in this child was not the result of birth asphyxia. Case closed.

Two years later, a different lawyer approached me about this case and asked me to review my opinion. By this time, new information had emerged that defined more clearly when an infant has suffered hypoxic-ischemic injury to the brain. The American College of Obstetricians and Gynecologists (ACOG) and the American Academy of Pediatrics (AAP) studied all the evidence at hand and concluded that an infant could have a brain injury if certain criteria were satisfied. These criteria, if satisfied, proved that the infant had suffered birth asphyxia of sufficient severity to cause an encephalopathy (brain disorder). Unfortunately, this condition was given the non-committal name of "neonatal encephalopathy." The criteria included: evidence of a "sentinel" event, an umbilical cord pH less than 7.00, and evidence of multiorgan injury as detected by laboratory studies of liver and kidney function. The rules of the game had changed.

I agreed to review the case and concluded this time that yes, there had been a neonatal encephalopathy as defined by the new criteria and, therefore, the case could be defended as a result of birth asphyxia. The plaintiff attorney and I reviewed carefully all the details of the case and how we could justify my opinion reversal. This would not be an easy task and the defense would be ready to attack with gusto the shifting expert witness. The meeting between the plaintiff and the defense was not pleasant. "Doctor, did you not give an expert opinion at one time that the client's cerebral palsy was *not* the result of birth asphyxia?" "Doctor, will you explain how you arrived at that conclusion?" "Doctor, you have recently reversed your opinion and contradicted yourself in this case. Please explain why you changed your opinion." I began by explaining that medicine is not an exact science and that progress comes from new studies and discoveries. The idea that malaria was caused by bad airs or miasmas dominated medical thinking until Laveran discovered that it was caused by a parasite transmitted by mosquitoes. Tuberculosis was caused by lack of good ventilation and nutrition until Koch identified the tuberculosis bacillus. Epilepsy was the result of possession by the devil until Hans Berger demonstrated abnormal brain waves in epileptic patients. The new definition of neonatal encephalopathy allowed for the previous untenable position to be changed. As simple as that! The case was settled once more.

Some pediatric neurologists like to offer their services as expert witnesses and others do not. Recent participation in a controversial case of vaccination-induced encephalopathy incriminated the expert witness as unreliable and dishonest. The motives of an expert witness who receives payment for his involvement in a legal case has been compared to a physician who prescribes a medication after receiving gifts from a pharmaceutical representative. Not all expert witnesses are motivated by remunerative factors. Some find justification in using their knowledge to benefit a doctor falsely accused or a patient victim of an error in judgment by a doctor or a hospital. I would like to think that as an expert witness I belonged to the latter group.

American College of Obstetricians and Gynecologists/American Academy of Pediatrics: *Neonatal Encephalopathy and Cerebral Palsy. Defining the Pathogenesis and Pathophysiology.* Washington, D.C., 2003.

Nelson KB, Ellenberg JH: Antecedents of cerebral palsy. Multivariate analysis of risk factors. *New England Journal of Medicine* 1986; 315: 81-6.

44

EMI SCAN

The new technology finally arrived in the United States from the U.K. in 1975. This was the first EMI scan that would allow visualization of the brain without need for invasive procedures. Prior to that, the only way for neurologists to look at the brain was to inject air (pneumoencephalogram) or contrast media (cysternography) into the spinal canal or into the cerebrovascular circulation (angiogram) to see if the ventricles were enlarged or if a mass displaced structures sufficiently to allow detection by conventional x-rays. Needless to say, these complicated procedures were reserved only for advanced cases when surgical intervention was inevitable.

A major advance using ultrasound permitted visualization of the neonatal brain while the anterior fontanelle was open. This allowed assessment of enlargement of the ventricles and the presence of intracranial hemorrhages. However, once the anterior fontanelle (soft spot) closed (usually by eighteen months of age), the cranium once again became the rigid box that guarded its secrets zealously. Clinicians became adept at interpreting signs and symptoms and a detailed neurological examination was the only key available to open this staunch defender of the brain it enclosed. That is, until the advent of the EMI scan.

The designation EMI scan has been replaced since by what is now known as CT scan. CT or computed tomography (also called CAT or computed axial tomography at the beginning) was developed applying computer technology to maximize the information obtained from x-ray studies. Before then, an x-ray study (or radiograph) only provided images of bone; other tissues were mostly radiolucent except for air and fat, which were easily detected. For more than half a century, conventional x-ray studies played an important role in diagnostic radiology. But still the brain and other organs could not be visualized directly until CT technology arrived.

As I recall, the anecdotal reports stated that Godfrey Hounsfield (1919-2004), who received the Nobel prize in 1970 for his development of CT, was a British government employee who was working on a project to find a way to see through thick walls and gather valuable intelligence data. His daughter was involved in an equestrian accident and suffered a traumatic head injury severe enough to induce coma. Her father agonized over the doctors' inability to detect if there was brain swelling, bleeding or other type of injury to help determine prognosis. Using his knowledge of physics and x-rays, he devised a computerized method of amplifying the information obtained from routine x-ray studies of the head so that previously undetected differences in soft-tissue organs, some more radiopaque and some more radiolucent, could be translated into a meaningful image of the brain. The technology was developed commercially by EMI (Electrical and Musical Industries), the same company that recorded the Beatles' music. Although initially the images were coarse due to the reduced number of pixels possible for each image, nevertheless the first non-invasive visualization of the brain was an incredible experience for us. One of the first studies in our patients was to detect tuberous sclerosis, a neurocutaneous disorder with subependymal glial nodules (benign tumors) in the brain. The latter appeared unmistakably as calcified lesions in the EMI scan. The key to opening the secret box had been found.

The leap from computed tomography to magnetic resonance (MR) took only a few years. Not only did MR improve the quality of the images but also avoided the exposure of ionizing radiation to children. The newer technology capitalized on the concept that all our tissues have water in different amounts or concentrations. The brain, for example, is about 80 percent water, the grey matter having more than the white matter. This small difference is sufficient for MR to render clear images of both. The technology uses magnetic resonance. A powerful magnet polarizes or aligns all the water molecules in the same direction and then spins these. The rate of spinning depends on the density and water concentration of each tissue. The resonance energy is then detected and converted into superb images by sophisticated computer programs. Each MR study of the brain may provide as many as one thousand separate images.

The advances in neuroimaging in the last century have been outstanding. The joke in medical centers was that with MR there was no longer a need for neurologists. However, as in many other endeavors, the good comes with the bad. Patients demand now MR studies for simple tension-type headaches or migraine. Physicians order MR because of medicolegal apprehension. These unnecessary tests add to the cost of health care. A thorough neurological examination will still answer most questions about diagnosis, treatment and prognosis. CT and MR should only be used to confirm clinical suspicions and not to screen for possible neurological disorders.

Hounsfield's parental concern about his daughter's brain translated into technological advances that benefited mankind. Who can imagine what even more outstanding discoveries in the future may change completely the way we practice medicine today? As for me, I have seen enough in the last fifty years to satisfy my own curiosity.

45

CNS

For a pediatric neurologist, CNS has two important meanings: central nervous system and Child Neurology Society, the main association of child neurologists in the United States.

As I recall, the roots of the Child Neurology Society started in the upper Midwest, when child neurologists from Minnesota, Iowa, Wisconsin and Michigan began meeting once a year to share interesting cases. Many of the meetings took place in a lodge near the Mississippi River. The meetings were collegial and only the residents and fellows attending were apprehensive, since they were required to present a paper. The strict scrutiny by Robert Landau was enough to unnerve even the most confident presenter. He would interrupt at any moment and challenge anything that had been said. Later, Landau would challenge his colleagues with a series of papers in the journal *Neurology* titled "Neuromyths" in which he would revel at dispelling many things we had accepted before as the truth. We all admired but feared this undaunted warrior. On a memorable occasion, one of the junior presenters came prepared. As soon as Dr. Landau interrupted him to challenge what he had just said, he pulled a toy gun from his pocket, pulled the trigger and a red flag with the word "BANG!" popped out. Even Dr. Landau had to laugh and it was the only time I ever saw anyone win an argument with him.

As the membership of the group increased, rumors began to circulate that some were sympathetic to forming a separate society from the American Academy of Neurology. The latter, although also headquartered in the upper Midwest, had become too big and the small group of child neurologists felt that they had become "lost" among the thousands of members of the Academy. An informal census showed that the majority did not favor a separatist movement. Nevertheless, at an informal meeting in La Crosse, Wisconsin, that included Bill Bell, Ray Chun, George Wolcott, Manny Gomez, Paul Dyken, Dick Allen and Frank Swaiman, it was agreed to formally create an association of child neurologists: the Child Neurology Society. There was initially, as mentioned, opposition to this move and later resentment. But slowly and surely, the CNS began to grow and at each annual meeting the attendance increased accordingly.

Child neurologists from the three Virginia medical schools (University of Virginia, Medical College of Virginia and Eastern Virginia Medical School) had been meeting every year at Colonial Williamsburg for a week-end of educational and social activities organized by Jimmy Etheridge, neurology chairman at Eastern Virginia Medical School. We decided to ask the CNS if we could have the next annual meeting in Williamsburg with the support of the three medical schools. The CNS approved the venue and members of the three medical schools worked together to make this a memorable meeting. The logistics of transporting members from airports in Washington, D.C., Richmond and Norfolk taxed our funds and energy, but all went well. The Hower Award for an outstanding child neurologist was given to Betty Banker and she was introduced by her husband, Maurice Victor, at the evening banquet. As the lights were dimmed and a procession of servers entered the banquet room with flaming plates of baked Alaska, the convened group broke into an enthusiastic applause. The 350 members who attended the meeting in Williamsburg were treated to something very special that evening.

The CNS has continued to grow and now lists about 1,200 members. This growth was fostered by well-chosen leaders and the untiring help of Mary Currey, the executive secretary, who answered all questions and solved all problems. However, child neurology as a specialty is in grave danger. It is the only pediatric subspecialty that has declined rather than grown in numbers. This phenomenon has resulted in an insufficient number of available child neurologists and at least forty positions remain unfilled at present, mainly in academic centers.

The main reason for the decline in interest by students and residents in child neurology as a specialty can be traced, I believe, to the ill-advised decision by the American Academy of Pediatrics that neurology was not an obligatory rotation by trainees in pediatrics. Why did they not choose cardiology or infectious diseases instead? About 40 percent of all patients seen by pediatricians have neurological problems. Not only did this decision stimulate students and residents to choose other specialties, but made pediatricians uneasy about handling neurological problems since their training lacked any exposure to neurology. As I realized the dire consequences of this decision, I wrote to Thomas Aceto, Jr., expressing my great concern about the consequences of this action. The answer was already known: the Academy and Board of Pediatrics, both decided that developmental pediatrics would provide all a pediatrician needed to know about neurology. Although, not voiced outright, some of us felt that we were penalized for not coming under the aegis of pediatrics (American

Academy of Pediatrics) and had chosen to align ourselves with neurology (American Academy of Neurology and Psychiatry).

The attrition of child neurology as a pediatric subspecialty is of much concern. Something drastic needs to be done to reverse the declining trend of the past two decades. We need to expose students and residents to child neurology early in their training so that child neurology can be included in their ultimate career choices. All we need is to attract one or two students each year and mentor them all the way until they become child neurologists. This means showing our clinical skills and knowledge as early as possible during their clinical training.

The training programs in child neurology also need to be streamlined. There is no need for the child neurology fellow to spend a whole year in adult neurology. Child and adult neurology are as different as night and day. If possible, the number of years required to complete child neurology training should be reduced. Why should we be boarded in *both* pediatrics and pediatric neurology? We only need one board in child neurology. The creation of a separate board in child neurology is the next logical step in the streamlining process. Just as the Child Neurology Society was created to give us autonomy, so also the creation of a Board of Child Neurology is necessary to help us regain our status as a bona fide subspecialty.

Swaiman KF: The organization of the Child Neurology Society: a personal view. *Pediatric Neurology* 1996; 15: 9-16.

46

DENDRITES AND SPINES

My old edition of the Merriam-Webster's Collegiate Dictionary defines a hypothesis as a tentative assumption in order to draw out and tests its logical or empirical consequences. A hypothesis implies insufficient evidence to provide more than a tentative explanation, while a theory implies a greater range of evidence and greater likelihood of truth. Hence, I wish to take licensure to present some ideas and assumptions formulated over the years about brain function.

Since I was young enough to meditate about mundane things such as why ants work in a colony with pre-assigned tasks for workers, warriors, drones, etc., all for the common good, or why polar bears hibernate, I have became convinced that nature evolves according to Darwinian principles and what we have at present represents its most refined and perfected examples of living things, including plants and animals. As such, the human brain represents the most sophisticated of nature's achievements to the extent that humans are the dominant species and the survival or destruction of our planet rests wholly in our hands.

The human brain weighs about 1,400 grams (three pounds) and contains approximately 20 billion (20,000,000,000 or 20×10^9) neurons (nerve cells) interconnected by some 70 trillion (70,000,000,000,000 or 70×10^{12}, or about 3,500 per neuron) connections called synapses. The cortex (also called gray matter because of its grayish appearance) is a thin ribbon (1.5 to 4.5 mm thick) on the surface of the brain where most neurons reside. In order to accommodate this inordinate large number of cells, the cortex has evolved from a flat surface to one consisting of many folds (gyri) separated by troughs (sulci). This most astute development allows for all these neurons to fit within the relatively small protective enclosure of the skull. Lacking this gyration process, our brain would look more like a pizza box measuring about half a meter (1.5 feet) on each side for a total surface area of almost 0.3 square meter (about 2.5 square feet), and we would appear to alien visitors as "kite-heads" bumping into each other and unable to see the stage well when seated behind each other in a movie-house or football stadium.

Even more astonishing, the twenty billion neurons are located in orderly layers which differ somewhat from region to region. Korbinian Brödmann (1868-1918), a German neurologist, was able to classify the brain into more than fifty separate areas according to the cytoarchitectonic (cell organization into layers) appearance under the microscope of these layers and assigned a different function to each. Although today such a rigid classification based on anatomical characteristics is not as popular as it once was, neurosurgeons and pathologists still have practical applications for Brödmann's classification. The different speech, auditory, memory, motor and sensory areas become important during surgical removal of tumors or epileptic tissue and are mapped in detail to prevent loss of vital brain functions.

One of the most amazing stages in brain development occurs towards the end of the first trimester when all the neurons start a pre-determined journey from the germinal matrix zone deep in the middle of the brain.

Each neuron is given an "order" to reach a specific target and elongated processes (fibers) from glial cells serve as bridges to guide each neuron to reach the assigned destination. This process has been captured in vivo and one can see the neurons advance with worm-like movements along the glial pathways. The incredible part of all this is that, at least in most of us, this complex mechanism goes on without a glitch. Each neuron is able to reach the end of its journey and pre-assigned location in our brain, guided by the almost infallible glial travel agency and its competent tour guides.

Nevertheless, errors do occur during neuronal migration. When these happen, the results may be intellectual impairment and seizures. The cortex in these cases does not show the orderly placement or laminar organization that characterizes the normal brain. The cortex is now thicker, smoother, more or less convoluted, and the component neurons are not distributed in uniform layers but appear to be in the wrong places and the size and shape of the neurons may be distorted. Neuropathologists recognized these abnormalities many years ago and called these cortical dysplasias. The advent of modern neuroimaging techniques, especially MRI, allowed for the recognition of these abnormalities in living patients. These were now grouped under the term neuronal migration disorders, among which lissencephaly (smooth brain), pachygyria (thick brain), polymicrogyria (many small folds), shizencephaly (split brain) and heterotopias (misplaced brain) are only a few of the numerous examples encountered in our clinics. Classification of these disorders is no easy task. A pediatric neurologist at the University of Chicago, Bill Dobyns, and a neuroradiologist from the University of California in San Francisco, A. James Barkovitch, have presented a classification of neuronal migration disorders and periodically update this. The human brain is, indeed, a marvelous and complex creation but still shrouded in mystery and, for the most part, only poorly understood.

An interesting question that a neurologist or neuroscientist may ask is: "Why do we dream?" Why do we spend one third of our lives in what seems an unproductive state during which nothing palpable is accomplished? Most persons require eight hours of sleep per day, although some persons, like Napoleon, claimed that they need only four hours of sleep. Other persons may sleep excessively and have a genetic disorder called narcolepsy. These tend to fall asleep anytime, anywhere. In addition, narcolepsy may exhibit cataplexy, a state of paralysis brought on by sudden fright or even laughter without any alteration in the level of consciousness. Even certain animals such as beagles and goats may exhibit cataplexy when they bark or become frightened.

During sleep, we dream. Some dreams are vivid and frightening, while others are pleasant and even euphoric. For millennia, different cultures have ascribed to dreams a spiritual component and the interpretations of dreams have resulted in predicting the future or, more practical, winning lottery numbers. Dreams may be especially distressing and in children pavor nocturnus (night terrors) are commonly associated with frightening figures from horror movies and, before the advent of television, reading scary stories such as Grimm's fairy tales.

The scientific study of sleep began with the development of the electroencephalogram (EEG) by a German psychiatrist, Hans Berger (1873-1941). Despite the exigencies of the war, Berger was able to continue his quest of recording the electrical activity of the brain. This was not an easy task, as he had to amplify the feeble electrical discharges a million times for these to be recorded by sensitive pens on paper. At the same time, Berger had to block out the interference caused by surrounding electrical equipment, otherwise the brain wave recordings were impossible to interpret. Berger may have been the first person to see different brain waves during sleep. This led to the recognition that brain waves change during sleep and these can be classified into four or five different stages, from stage 1 (drowsy) all the way to stages 3-4 (deep sleep). More importantly, the deepest stage of sleep was accompanied by rapid-eye movements and restlessness (hence named REM sleep). Soon it was established that most dreams occur during REM sleep. Despite the development of sleep laboratories, sleep research studies and sleep disorders as a neurological subspecialty, we still don't know why we sleep. We do know that the brain needs sleep to rest, otherwise the next morning will find us tired, both physically and mentally. Unfortunately, Berger, who was emeritus professor of psychology, died from suicide without receiving the recognition he deserved for his great discovery.

During the wake state, the brain receives an unconceivable large number of messages or stimuli from all the receptors that populate our five senses. These messages convey to us what is happening in the outside world. The information is then processed immediately so that important decisions can be made necessary to respond appropriately, be it a conversation, a sudden unexpected danger or an inspiring moment. It is impossible for any computer to process and store this amount of information every second, every minute, every hour of our wake existence. There has to be a mechanism by which the brain "cleanses" or "detoxifies" itself from useless information it will no longer need after a certain amount of time has elapsed. The computer (our brain), then shuts down and begins the process of deleting all that information it no longer needs. The process must be effective and cleans the brain so that next day it can function effectively and process new information without glitches. Were it not for this renewal activity during sleep, our brain would become overloaded and "implode" for lack of needed memory space. The brain is the most sophisticated computer known. No computer can survive and function effectively for seven or eight decades without a support mechanism designed to maintain it fresh and ready to go on the next day. Since the number of synapses is relatively fixed after a certain age, it makes sense to think that these connections are renewed each day, just as a teacher erases the blackboard so that next day it can be used again to teach new things to the students. Without the daily cleansing, the blackboard would become cluttered, without the necessary space to jot down new information.

Not long ago, I was invited to participate in a symposium on ADHD to be held in Madrid and given the choice to select any subject associated with ADHD. Unwittingly, I decided to talk about the "neurological examination in ADHD," realizing only too late that there was little of interest I could discuss. However, in searching the literature I found a study recently done at NIH by Philip Shaw and his colleagues on ADHD with (to me) startling findings. Children with ADHD were found to differ from normal controls in that they developed a thicker cerebral cortex and achieved this at a later age than controls (10.5 vs 7.5 years). After that, the cortex appeared to gradually reduce its thickness. I say startling because we are accustomed to finding less and fewer of whatever we are measuring in patients affected by brain disorders. This study found there was *more* of something in ADHD patients. This excess, for example, could be more dendritic spines and connections (synapses) than necessary between neurons in ADHD children.

As the brain develops, these connections between neurons may be visualized and even quantified by special staining of the axons and dendrites that interconnect neurons. The process is named dendritic arborization and appears to reach a peak at about two years of age, when the maturational processes of the brain are thought to reach completion. However, the studies at NIH have shown that the brain continues to make these connections until about age seven years, after which the number of synapses is reduced to a more manageable number (whatever that number is). In other words, the brain continues to increase the network of connections in excess of what it will eventually need, until it stops and then selectively reduces the number to a more practical number to meet its physiological needs.

Neuropsychologists and linguists have observed that a child is able to learn a different language more easily than an adult. The ability to speak a second (third or fourth) language without a foreign accent is the prerogative of a young person until the age of about six years. After that, the circuits are fixed and the ear cannot distinguish the fine nuances of one language from another. This means that the younger brain is more adaptable, or as is more technically explained, has more plasticity. Plasticity is beneficial also when a child has a stroke, for example, since the child may recover sooner or better than an adult. In other words, the child's brain is able to adapt and make changes more easily than the adult or "fixed" brain.   An excess abundance of synapses between neurons may be an important component of this linguistic or neurologic recovery adaptability.

An excess number of synapses could also explain ADHD. Too many interconnections facilitate the dissemination of external stimuli, such as visual, auditory, tactile, etc., messages that cannot be filtered selectively because there are too many available connections. As the NIH studies showed, ADHD brains have too many connections (synapses) and these undermine the ability to stay focused and on task. Too many unnecessary impulses generate distractibility and impulsivity, two important diagnostic components of ADHD.

There is also, at least in my mind, some resemblance between autism and ADHD. Autism is characterized by delayed communication (see above about children's ability to learn languages), defective interpersonal or social interactions and stereotyped repetitive activities such as rocking movements, head banging, etc. Autistic children are commonly hyperactive, with short attention spans, and impulsive. They are unable to engage in meaningful play by themselves or with other children. Although autism and ADHD are two distinct separate disorders, a similar mechanism may underlie both deficiencies. As in ADHD, if autism were associated with too many synapses, the ability to develop communication and social skills would be impaired. Since in the majority of autistic children conventional studies such as EEGs, CT and MRI neuroimaging fail to show any abnormality, the aberrant brain function in these conditions must either reside at a sub-microscopic or chemical (neurotransmitter) level.

V.S. Ramachandran, a provocative and brilliant neuroscientist, has resolved some of the most challenging and complex neurological problems. Upper limb amputees suffer from a distressing condition called "phantom-limb pain." Although the arm is no longer there, the brain continues to recognize its presence and receives pain signals when it cannot move or change position of the phantom limb. The pain is so distressing that some patients end their misery by suicide. Ramachandran fooled the brain by using a mirror to reflect movement from the unaffected limb and thus create the illusion that the phantom limb was moving and changing position when in reality this was occurring on the contralateral side. The rate of cure and improvement was unprecedented.

Ramachandran thinks that some psychiatric conditions may represent abnormal connections between separate regions of the brain with different functions. Schizophrenia with hallucinations, multiple personality disorders, bipolar behaviors, may be explained physiologically by abnormal connections (synapses) between unrelated brain regions. These novel ideas may open new horizons in the research to solve neurological and psychiatric disorders.

My hypothesis is simple. I believe that disorders such as ADHD and autism have a similar underlying pathophysiological mechanism: too many synapses. The brain provides itself with an excess of synapses in early and late childhood to accommodate for the acquisition of complex functions such as learning a language and social skills. Once these important functions are acquired, the brain then reduces the number of synapses to a more reasonable quantity. ADHD and autism develop when this reduction of synapses process fails or is disrupted. Both disorders have a similar underlying basic mechanism of too many interneuronal connections. Learning and storing information are impaired due to too many dendritic spines and synapses. Instead of focusing on a specific task, the brain is distracted by too many other messages coming in from outside and facilitated by an overabundance of circuits and connections. The result is too many distractions that keep interrupting the learning process. Hyperactivity is the response to too many stimuli from outside without proper screening or selectivity. In autism, the intricate tasks of language and communication are not properly learned because the synapses necessary to facilitate the process of language development are exhausted by age two years due to a lack of renovation mainly during sleep. The analogy would be trying to download a new program in our computer when there is insufficient memory left in the hard disk to accommodate it. The autistic brain is no longer able to process new information necessary to learn to speak, develop imaginative play or to interpret facial expressions and body language required for social interaction. It is perhaps no coincidence that autism is usually not recognized or diagnosed until about the age two years. This may be the lapse of time required to overload all of the available connections in the brain when there is no effective renewal system. Thus, the important tools needed to function well in society are not available and the brain is unable to complete its maturational process.

Many years ago, a pediatric neurologist at NIH, Karin Nelson, was able to demonstrate that most children with cerebral palsy are not the due to birth asphyxia or poor obstetrical techniques. Instead, many are due to interruptions in the process of neuronal migration at the end of the first trimester so that interconnections between neurons are severely impaired. Similarly, a defect in maturational processes of dendritic spines and synapses may explain disorders such as ADHD and autism. Since Ramón y Cajal's (1852-1934) first anatomical description of spines (*espinas* or thorns) in 1891, we know little about what controls the formation, interconnections and elimination of dendritic spines. More research and studies in this neglected area may provide important clues to a better understanding of such ADHD, autism and other childhood neurological disorders.

Barkovich AJ, Guerrini R, Kuzniecky RI, Jackson GD, Dobyns WB: A developmental and genetic classification for malformations of cortical development: update 2012. *Brain* 2012; 135 (Part 5): 1348-1369.

Hutsler JJ, Zhang H: Increased dendritic spine densities on cortical projection neurons in autism spectrum disorders. *Brain Research* 2010; 1309: 83-94

Ramachandran VS, Blakeslee S: *Phantoms in the Brain. Probing the Mysteries of the Human Mind.* New York: Harper Perennial, 1998.

Shaw P, Eckstrand K, Sharp W, et al: Attention-deficit/ hyperactivity disorder is characterized by a delay in cortical maturation. *Proceedings National Academy of Sciences U.S.A.* 2007; 104: 19649-19654.

INDEX

Aceto, Jr., Thomas, 233
Acute life threatening
  event (ALTE), 21
Ada, Oklahoma, v
Adipic acid, 35-7
Aedes egypti, 60,68
Aflatoxins, 4,7-8
Agalychnis callidrys, 204
Agramonte, Aristides, 61,63
Albinism, 89-92
Alice-in-Wonderland
  syndrome, 160
Allen, Dick, 232
Alopecia areata, 191
*American Journal of Diseases
  of Children*, 28
*American Journal of Tropical
  Medicine & Hygiene*, 100
Amitriptyline, 109
Amodiaquine, 98-100,105
Amyloidosis, 46
Ancon Hospital, 183,212
Ancylostoma duodenale, 72
Anopheles albimanus, 93,183
Anticonvulsant, 15,117-8,
  155
Antiepileptic drugs, 117
Aposematism, 204
Arachnoid cyst, 179
Arosemena, Ascanio, 188
Asperger syndrome, 169
Aspergillus flavus, 4
Aspirin, 10,144,163
Attention deficit hyperactivity
  disorder (ADHD), 240-5
Auras, migraine, 161-2

Autism, 49,139,172,190,
  242-5
Autism spectrum disorder
  (ASD), 169,242-5
Autonomic disorder, 153-4
Autonomic nervous system,
  152-4
Autopsy, chemical, 21-25

Babinski, Josef, 115
*Bacille Calmette-
  Guérin* (BCG), 75-9
Bacillus icteroides, 61
Banker, Betty, 232
Barkovitch, James, 237
Batten, Fred, 89,147
Batten's disease, 147-9
Bell, Bill, 232
Bell, Joseph, 199
Benign paroxysmal positional
  vertigo (BPPV), 158
Benign paroxysmal vertigo
  (BPV), 158-60
Berger, Hans, 226,238-9
Biblioteca Nacional, 207
Birth asphyxia, 126,224-
  5,238-9,244
Bolivian hemorrhagic
  fever, 52
Bouchama, Abderrezak, 144
Brain death, 121-3
Brain dendrites, 235,241
Brain spines, 235,241,243-4
Brödmann, Korbinian, 236
Butantán Institute, 42-3

Calomys callosus, 52
Canal Zone, v,41,52,77-
  8,87,184-8,209-10,212
Cannibalism, 135
Carroll, James, 61-3,67

Carroll, Lewis
(Charles Dodgson), 160
Cataplexy, 173,238
Cerebral palsy, 126,172,174,
224-5,244
Ceroid, 147-9
Chaillé, Stanford, 60
Charcot, Jean-Martin, 115,
165
Chaulmoogra oil, 46
Child Neurology Society
(CNS), 231-3
Chlordane, 93-4
Chloroquine, 98,105
Cholesterol granuloma, 179-
80
Chrysomia marcellaria, 87
Chun, Ray, 232
Chytridiomycosis, 204
Clara Maass Medical
Center, 68
Clendening History of
Medicine Library, vi,vii
Clinicopathological
conference (CPC), 21-2,151
Coco Solo Hospital, 41,52,
98-9
Communicable Disease
Center (CDC), 5,52
Computed tomography
(CT), 5,76,228-9
Conan Doyle, Sir Arthur, 199
Concussion, 107-9
Cortical dysplasia, 237
Costa Rica, v,44,94,104,126,
163,204,207
Crenner, Christopher, vi
Critchley, Macdonald, 216
Currey, Mary, 233

Darling, Samuel Taylor, vi,
56,72,104,183-4,209-13

D.D.T., 93-4
Dendrites, 235,241
Department of History and
Philosophy of Medicine, vi
Department of Pediatrics,
vi,55
Dermatobia hominis, 85
Diphtheria, 46-9
Discrimination, Canal Zone,
186
Dobyns, Bill, 237
Dreams, 238-9
Duchenne, Guillaume
Benjamin Amand de
Boulogne, 165
Duchenne muscular
dystrophy (DMD), 165
Duffin, Jacalyn, 178
Dyck, Peter, 154
Dyken, Paul, 148,232

Eastern Virginia Medical
School (EVMS), 195,232
Electroencephalogram (EEG),
18,114,117,123,136,152,
169,174-5,238,242
Ellefson, Ralph, 7,9
Ellenberg, Jonas, 224
EMI scan, 227-9
Engle, Andrew, 154
Epilepsy, 114-5,226
Etheridge, Jimmy, 232
Ethylmalonic acid, 36
Expert witness, 28,219-26

Fer-de-lance, 41
Fildes, Sir Luke, iv
Finlay, Carlos, 59-63
Fishman, Marvin, 140
Fleas, 94
Fore, 135
Frenkel, Jack, 55-6

Freud, Sigmund, 115

Gajdusek, Carleton, 135-6
Galactosemia, 24
Gantry, Elmer, 177
Garrod, Sir Archibald, 89
Gas chromatography (GC),
  35,170,194-5
Gastaut, Henri, 154
Gawande, Atul, vi,216
Ghon complex, 76-7
Gilles de la Tourette,
  Georges, 115,173
Glomerulonephritis, acute,
  82-3
Glycine receptor, 175
Gold roll employees, 186
Gomez, Manuel R., v,232
Gorgas Hospital, v,41,43,46,
  52,76,183-5,209,211-2
Gorgas Memorial Laboratory,
  100
Gorgas, William, 56,98,105,
  183,209,211
Gowers, William, 154,165
Grocott, Robert, 43
Gusanillo, 33

Hair abnormalities, 189-91
Hallpike-Turner maneuver,
  158
Havana, Cuba, 60-3,66,68
Heatstroke, 29,143-4
Hejazi, Nadia, 175
Hemorrhagic shock, 27,29
Hermetia illucens, 86
Histoplasmosis, vi,43,56,183,
  210-2
Holmes, Fred, vii
Holmes, Grace, vii
Holmes, Sherlock, 47,199
Homocystinuria, 24

Hookworm, 71-3,211
Hounsfield, Godfrey, 228,
  230
Humphreys, Margaret, 59
Hyperekplexia, 173-5
Hyperthermia, 13,144-5
Hypotonia, 126,128,169
Hypoxic-ischemic
  encephalopathy, 174,223,
  225

Imam, 118,121
Impetigo, 53,81-3,85
Inborn errors of metabolism
  (IEM), 4,24,89,129,132,
  190,194-5
Index Medicus, 42,208
Indirect immunofluorescent
  antibody test (IFAT), 53
Influenza, 5,7
Isthmian Canal Commission
  (ICC), 105,186,213

Jackson, Sir Hughlings,
  117,154
Jakob-Creutzfeldt disease,
  136
Jell-O®, 35-7
Johnson, Chet, vi
Johnson, George, 3
Johnson, Karl, 52
*Journal of the American
  Medical Association*, 56
*Journal of Inherited
  Metabolic Diseases*, 36

Kanner, Leo, 169
Kansas University Medical
  Center (KUMC), vii,55
Kohl, 32
Kuna Indians, 88,90-2
Kuru, 135-7

Lancet, 3,4,27-8,55,89
Landau, Robert, 231
Las Animas Hospital, 62-65, 67-8
Laveran, Alphonse, 97,226
Lazear, Jesse, 61-2,67
Lead poisoning, 31-3
Leão, cortical depression of, 162
Leigh's disease, 130-2
Leprosy, 46
Lesseps, Ferdinand de, 59,209
Lipofuscin, 147-9
Little, Rich, 201
Littlejohn, Henry, 199
Low, Phillip, 154

Maass, Clara, vii,59,63-8
Maass, Sophia, 66
Magnetic resonance imaging (MRI), 5,76,107, 128,131,161-2,169,179-80,237,242
Malaria, 59,68,93,97-100,104-5,125,144,183, 209,211,226
Mantoux test, 75-7
Maria Chiquita, 41
Mass spectrometry (MS), 24,35,170,194-5
Mayo Clinic, v,6,154
Mayo Clinic Proceedings, 6,8,209
Mayo Medical Laboratories, 25-6
Medium chain acyl CoA deficiency (MCAD), 4
Metamorphopsia, 160
Methemoglobinemia, 13-5
Methylene blue, 13,52

Mézerville, Esther de, 207
Miasmas, 59,60-1,68,97,125
Middle America Research Unit (MARU), 52-3
Migraine, 103-4,160-4,229
Migraine, abdominal, 159
Migraine, acute confusional, 161
Migraine equivalents, 160-1
Migraine, treatment, 162-3
Miracles, 177-8
Mitochondria, 4,10,37,129-33
Mola, 90-1
Monilethrix, 190
Moon children, 89,90
Mucopolysaccharidosis, 24
Münchhausen, 17-8
Münchhausen by proxy, 15,17-8
Myasis, 85-6
Myoglobinuria, 129,131, 133,145

Narcolepsy, 173,238
National Collaborative Perinatal Project (NCPP), 224
Necator americanus, 72
Nelson, Karin, 224,244
Neonatal encephalopathy, 225-6
Neurology (Journal), 231
Neuronal ceroid-lipofuscinosis (NCL), 147-9
Newborn screening, 23-4
New England Journal of Medicine, 21,123,151,208, 221
Nicolle, Charles, 51,56
Night terrors (*pavor nocturnus*), 238

Nigua, 94-5
Nurses, in Spanish-American
  War, 65
Nystagmus, 91-2,158

Occupational Safety and
  Health Administration
  (OSHA), 33
Oklahoma University
  College of Medicine, v
On-Line Mendelian
  Inheritance In Man
  (OMIM), 131
Organic acids, 170-1,196
Organic acidurias, 170
Ornithine transcarbamylase
  (OTC) deficiency, 4
Osler, Sir William, 42-3

Palo Seco leper colony, 46
Panama, vi,31,41,43,46,48,
  52-3,56,59, 72,75-7,81-
  3,86,89-93,98,100,104-
  5,126,183-5,209-11
Panama Canal, vi,56,59,68,
  75,86,98-9,184-5
Panama Canal Zone,
  v,41,52,77-8,87,98,184-
  8,209-10,212
Panama riots, January 29,
  1964, 185
Panayiatoupoulos, C.P., 154
Peralta, Pauline, 52
Percussion hammers, 122,
  127,184
Pervasive developmental
  disorders (PDD), 169
Phantom limb pain, 242-3
Phenobarbital, 118
Phenylketonuria (PKU), 23
Phenytoin, 118-9
Pica, 31-33

Picado, Clodomiro, 44
Pili torti, 190
Pincus, Jonathan, 131
Piringer-Kuchinka, 54
Plasmodium falciparum,
  97,104
Pope John Paul II, 178
Pope Pius XII, 122
Postural orthostatic
  tachycardia syndrome
  (POTS), 153
Potter, Elizabeth, 82-3
Pregnancy test, toad, 203-5
Prions, 136
*Proceedings of the Canal
  Zone Medical Association*,
  86,212
Prosopagnosia, 199
Prusinger, Stanley, 136
Pseudoseizures, 114-5

Queen's Square, National
  Hospital for the Paralyzed
  and Epileptic, 127,147,154
Quinine, 98,100,103-5

Ragged red fibers, 131
Raggedy Ann, 125-6,128
Ramachandran, V.S., 242-3
Ramón y Cajal, Santiago,
  244
Reed, Walter, 45,61-4,67
Rett, Andreas, 139
Rett syndrome, 140-1
Revista Cultural La Lotería
  (Panama), vi
Revista de Neurología
  (Spain), 215
Reye, Douglas, 3,4,6,10
Reye-Johnson syndrome, 3
Reye syndrome, 3,5-10
Riley-Day syndrome, 153

Roberts, Oral, 177
Rockefeller Foundation, 71, 211-2
Rodríguez-Expósito, César, 68
Ross, Sir Ronald, 97
Royal Alexandra Hospital, 3
Ryanodine gene, 145

Sacks, Oliver, vi,199,216
Sanarelli, Giuseppe, 61
San Juan de Dios Hospital, 44
Sarcoglycanopathies, 167
Sarcoptes scabiei, 81
Scabies, 53,82-3
Scanlon, Gayle, 7
Seizures, 15,49,114-5,117-8,136,144,147,149,152,154-5,161,169,237
Selzer, Richard, vi,216
Shaken-baby syndrome, 18,108
Shaw, Philip, 240
Silver roll employees, 186
Skiagraphs, 76
Sleep, v,93,108,112,160, 188,238-40,244
Smallpox, 45
Snakebite, 41-4
Spanish-American War, 65-6
Spinal muscular atrophy (SMA), 167
Splenomegaly, 104-5
Spongiform encephalopathy, 136-7
Startle disease, 173-5
Status epilepticus, 117-9
Stegomyia, 60
Sternberg, George, 61,63-5
Stich, Virginia, 209-10,212-3
Stiles, Charles Wardell, 71

Sudden infant death syndrome (SIDS), 17,21, 175,196
Swaiman, Frank, 232
Sykes, Bryan, 130
Synapses, 199,236,240-4

Thiamine pyrophosphate inhibitor (TPP), 131
Toxoplasma gondii, 51
Toxoplasmosis, 51-6,85
Treponema pallidum, 144
Trichorrhexis nodosa, 190
Trichothiodystrophy, 190
Trichotillomania, 190-1
Trömner hammer, 127
Tuberculosis, 48,75-8, 210,226
Tuberous sclerosis, 199,229
Tunga penetrans, 94
Typhoid fever, 65
Üllrich-Turner Syndrome, 209
University Hospital, v,203

Vertebro-basilar migraine, 161
Vertigo, 157-9
Vertigo, benign paroxysmal (BPV), 158-9
Vertigo, benign paroxysmal positional (BPPV), 158
Victor, Maurice, 232
Vietnam War, 98,105
Villalobos, Nilo, 103-4
Vómito negro (black vomit), 59

Walton, Bryce, 52-6
Wear-and-tear pigments, 147
Werdnig-Hoffman disease, 167

Index 253

Wesleyan University, v
Whooping cough, 46
Williamsburg (VA), 232-3
Wisniewski, Kristina, 149
Wolcott, George, 232
Wood, Leonard, 63
World Health Organization
 (WHO), 71

Yeast hypothesis, 170-1
Yellow fever, vi,45,59-68,
 93,98,104,209
Yellow Fever Commission,
 60
Young, Rodolfo, 48

Zoghbi, Hoda, 140-1